CRPS AWARENESS

Moving against Pain

By

Sunny Boshoff

Published by Rightime Books 2010

Copyright ©
S. Boshoff and E. Lancaster 2010

Cartoon drawings – Sunny Boshoff
Layout – Peter Kováčik and Sonia Papajova
Cover Design – Elizabeth Lancaster, Sunny Boshoff and Victor David
Photographs, retouching and web design – Victor David
Logo Design – Phillip Bennett
Editors – Pamela Kozak and Elizabeth Lancaster

A catalogue record for this book is available from the British Library.

ISBN 978-0-9566360-0-3

Dedicated to my mom who is completely inspirational in the way she deals with the devastating effects of Parkinsons Disease and to my dear friend Shal who finally succumbed to breast cancer in January 2010.

Introduction

This book evolved from a diary which I began after a crush injury to my right hand. It started out as an exercise in teaching my left hand to write. After developing Complex Regional Syndrome (CRPS) it became an important daily ritual which helped to keep me somewhat sane during an excruciatingly painful year.

Having been diagnosed I quickly discovered the lack of awareness surrounding the condition. Very few in the medical profession had heard of CRPS. Some I encountered were very empathetic, but others appeared to think that my descriptions of the pain were either imagined or exaggerated.

I very soon realised that without access to the internet, those experiencing CRPS would find it very difficult to discover any information on it. There is very little in the way of printed material, other than in medical journals. This inspired the writing of the book.

I wanted to produce it in a way that it could be rested on the lap or on a table, without the reader having to hold the pages open, keeping in mind those with painful hands.

It is in chronological order in the hope that, both patients and health professionals who are not familiar with CRPS may benefit from the feedback and descriptions of my experience as the condition developed. The fact that I had disproportionate levels of pain seemed to alienate me at times, which was psychologically quite traumatic.

Without any health insurance I was extremely lucky to have been unconditionally supported, not only emotionally, but financially by my friends. This gave me the opportunity to explore and receive treatments that are as yet not funded by the NHS. CRPS is such an unknown condition at present in the UK, that I found, in general, pain medication and anti-depressants were pretty much all that was on offer for me.

Thankfully I was referred for Occupational Therapy in hand units. OT is accessible to everyone and it was in these units that I found understanding and a positive way forward.

Along with the Occupational Therapy which provided a strong foundation, I explored Acupuncture, Alexander Technique, Collateral Meridian Therapy, Osteopathy, Massage and Herbs.

I researched the history and philosophies of all of the above and discovered their common holistic approach. Their ethos is to instigate or re-invigorate a healthy whole system more able to deal with an illness or injury. In the case of OT there is particular attention paid to the psychological wellbeing of the patient, which is vital for those living with acute pain

It is important to say that I wanted to stick strictly to my experience and avoid including other methods which have been found to be successful, but of which I have no firsthand knowledge.

I would also like to say here and re-iterate all the way through the book that this is a record of how I dealt with my CRPS and anyone wishing to act on information in this book should discuss any decisions with a Health Professional.

I was keen to avoid relying heavily on pain medication which in the long term can create its own set of problems. This was a personal choice and is in no way intended to be judgemental. Because CRPS has such a range of breathtakingly painful symptoms, it is difficult not to succumb to powerful pain medication. My advice to anyone with CRPS is how important it is to try to keep moving your limb, try to see an Occupational Therapist as soon as and as often as possible and don't give up! Keep at it no matter how painful. That for me cannot be overstated.

Sunny Boshoff

Pain Relief Foundation

What Is Complex Regional Pain Syndrome (CRPS)?
Complex Regional Pain Syndrome Type I (CRPS I) is also known as Reflex Sympathetic Dystrophy (RSD) and Complex Regional Pain Syndrome Type II (CRPS II) is also known as Causalgia. The pain usually develops after an injury to an arm or leg. Only rarely are other areas affected.

CRPS I follows an injury to a limb such as a broken bone or even a minor sprain and CRPS II follows partial damage to a nerve in the limb. The symptoms are very similar. However, CRPS II is very rare.

The main symptom is pain in the arm or leg. The pain is often burning, sharp, stabbing or stinging, with tingling and numbness. In addition there is a range of other symptoms which can vary and change over time. Increased skin sensitivity (allodynia), increased sensitivity to pain (hyperalgesia), skin discolouration, swelling, stiffness, feelings of hot or cold, excessive or reduced sweating and changes to the hair, skin or nails. The pain and other symptoms usually spread beyond the site of the original injury.

Pain continues long after the original injury has healed. It is often severe and may get progressively worse. In mild cases the pain can last for weeks or months but in severe cases, when the limb is not used, it can last for years.

The skin may become over sensitive to light touch. Clothes brushing the skin, or a slight draught on the skin, is felt as severe pain. This is called allodynia and is common in CRPS.

Often there is difficulty moving the limb, together with weakness and sometimes tremors or jerking. In severe cases the limb can be fixed in one position.

In very severe cases there may be bone softening resulting in breaks. This is called osteopaenia. There can also be muscle atrophy (wasting) and in extreme cases muscle contracture.

What Causes CRPS?
CRPS is rare but can follow any injury.

CRPS Type I (RSD) follows an injury to the skin, muscle, ligaments, joints or bone at any site. The injury can be as a result of an accident or surgery. Most commonly it occurs after a bone is broken and immobilized with a splint or a sling, but can occur even after a minor sprain.

CRPS Type II (Causalgia) follows partial damage to a nerve in the arm or leg, such as from a gunshot wound or crush injury.

The cause of the prolonged pain and other symptoms is unknown. Changes in the way nerves send messages to the brain about pain may occur at the injury site. These changes may then lead to more changes in the nerves of the spinal cord and brain. All these changes are thought to play a role in causing and prolonging the condition.

CRPS may be prevented by ensuring that plaster casts and bandages are not too tight and that limbs are used as early as possible after injury.

Diagnosis

CRPS is not an easy condition to diagnose and often referral to a Pain Clinic is necessary for an accurate diagnosis. Other possible causes of pain need to be excluded first. There is usually an event such as an injury to a limb which causes damage or immobilization. There is continuous pain out of proportion to the original injury. Not everyone with CRPS has all the symptoms but they will have some of them. 70% have increased sensitivity to pain, 80-85% have abnormal changes in temperature (feelings of hot and cold), abnormal changes in skin colour, swelling or reduced movement, 50% have abnormal sweating, and 20% have weakness, tremor, increased muscle tone or changes in hair, nail or skin growth.

The Pain Specialist may carry out a series of tests – Quantitative Sensory Testing – to find out if there are any abnormalities of feeling in the affected area. They measure sensitivity to heat and cold, touch and pressure, skin blood flow rates and skin temperature.

Treatment

Early detection will help in managing the condition.

The primary aim of treatment is to restore full use to the painful limb, especially load bearing, e.g. standing and walking, despite the pain. Physiotherapy is a very effective treatment for CRPS. Intensive physiotherapy treatment and doing exercises taught by the physiotherapist at least twice a day are essential. Using the limb is very important.

Desensitization of the skin can help to counter the skin hypersensitivity. The skin is rubbed with a series of cloths of increasing coarseness, e.g. from silk to toweling. In addition alternate immersion in hot and cold baths can help temperature sensitivity

Drugs

There is no real evidence that drugs cure CRPS. But the pain may be partly relieved by drugs, which will help people to do the physiotherapy exercises. Common painkillers such as ibuprofen may help. Some patients may benefit from treatment with strong pain killers such as morphine. Tramadol is a milder drug, similar to morphine, which may sometimes be useful.

Antidepressant drugs such as amitriptyline or imipramine, originally developed to treat depression, can sometimes be useful for **nerve pain** (as in CRPS). They may cause side effects such as dry mouth, drowsiness, or constipation. It is often possible to get the right balance between side effects and pain relief so that they are of benefit.

Anticonvulsant drugs used for epilepsy treatment can also relieve **nerve pain**. Gabapentin or pregabalin (Lyrica®) are very useful drugs and Carbamazepine (Tegretol®) may help. You may have some side effects, such as tiredness and weight gain. These antidepressant and anticonvulsant drugs must be taken regularly for them to work and not just when the pain is bad. They can take up to 3 weeks to have an effect. They will probably need to be taken for a long time.

You may need to take more than one kind of drug. Your doctor will try to find the best combination for you.

Psychological Issues

People with CRPS may commonly develop depression and anxiety. Psychological support is very important. Pain Management Programmes may be useful in some people. Cognitive behavioural therapy (CBT) can be effective. The best treatment for CRPS is delivered by a multidisciplinary team involving doctors, occupational and physical therapists and psychologists.

Other Treatments

Transcutaneous Electrical Nerve Stimulation (TENS) may help some patients. This treatment, using electrodes placed on the painful area, causes a tingling sensation, which may reduce the pain.

Spinal cord stimulation (SCS) can be an effective treatment for CRPS in a few suitable people. An electrical stimulator is implanted under the skin and an electrode is placed next to the spinal cord. This treatment is only available in a few specialist centres, for suitable patients in whom all other treatments have been ineffective.

Nerve blocks. There is no evidence that these injections to the limb are an effective cure for CRPS. However, they may help enough so that physiotherapy can be done.

Mirror Visual Feedback. This treatment is still experimental, but has helped in some cases. A mirror is placed so that it reflects the opposite, unaffected limb, so that it looks as if the affected limb is normal. When the opposite limb is moved the person sees the affected limb move in the mirror. The affected limb can then also be felt to move. (This is called kinesthetic sensations.) If this is repeated many times it may lead to normal movement of the affected limb and reduction in pain.

Where To Get Help And Support

The British Pain Society, www.britishpainsociety.org
21 Portland Place, London W1B 1PY.
Can provide patient information leaflets such as: 'Understanding and Managing Pain: Information for Patients' and 'Spinal Cord Stimulation for Pain: Information for Patients'

The Pain relief Foundation is not responsible for the content of any information provided by another organization and does not endorse any product or service mentioned or advised by any other organization.

The material on these pages appears in a pamphlet which was published by the staff of the Pain Relief Foundation and endorsed by The Walton Centre Pain Team, Walton Centre for Neurology & Neurosurgery, Lower Lane, Liverpool, L9 7LJ, UK. **www.thewaltoncentre.co.uk**

The Pain Relief Foundation is a registered charity. If you found the content of these pages useful please consider donating to the Foundation. Every donation helps to fund research into the treatment of all chronic pain conditions.

Pamphlets are available from The Pain Relief Foundation, Clinical Sciences Centre, University Hospital Aintree, Lower Lane, Liverpool L9 7AL, UK.
Registered Charity No. 277732.
Tel. 0151 529 5820
Fax. 0151 529 5821
email: secretary@painrelieffoundation.org.uk

Other leaflets in the series:

Trigeminal Neuralgia	Phantom Limb Pain	Arthritis
Low back pain	Sciatica	Pain after Stroke
Shingles & PHN	Pain in Diabetes	Cancer Pain
Fibromyalgia	Headache	Opioids for chronic pain

Disclaimer: If you have a pain problem which needs treatment you must contact your own doctor. He can refer you to a pain clinic in your area. This leaflet is for information only and should not be treated as a substitute for the medical advice of your doctor. The Pain Relief Foundation cannot offer individual medical advice.

Copyright of The Pain Relief Foundation and is reproduced with their kind permission.

...the rattling of a newspaper, a breath of air, the step of another across the ward, the vibrations caused by a military band or the shock of the feet in walking, gives rise to increase of pain.

At last the patient grows hysterical, if we may use the only term which describes the facts. He walks carefully, carries the limb with the sound hand, is tremulous, nervous and has all kinds of expedients for lessening his pain.

S. Weir Mitchell – On Causalgia (CRPS)
Recorded during The American Civil War 1861–1865
Injuries of Nerves and their Consequences.
Published by
J.R. Lippincott & Co 1872

The Crush and The Diary

On Friday 13th July 2007 my friend Shal drove into her garage and parked. We then tried to unload a large garden pot from the back seat of her convertible mini. The pot had no handles and weighing about 80 lbs was quite difficult to manoeuvre. I had pushed the driver's seat forward and with one foot in the car I lifted the underneath of the pot while Shal lifted it from above. All was good and we got it over the edge of the car, but as I tried to step out my foot caught on the seat belt and I felt myself being pulled to the ground. This left poor Shal trying to keep a grip onto the sides of the pot.

Because it was quite dark in the garage it added to the confusion of what happened next. I heard her let out a shriek and I found myself on the floor on both hands and knees. In that flash, I knew that I should be afraid, that something dangerous was happening.

Then I just felt the pot crash down on my right hand with a sickening crunch, that I had no doubt was the sound of my bones being crushed.

The whole agenda changed as we realised that my hand was quite badly injured. We both knew that I had to get to hospital as soon as possible. It was a warm summer day and as we reversed out of the garage into the sunshine I felt like I was in a vacuum and Shal's voice as she spoke gently to me sounded far away. I knew I had to stay calm.

A therapeutic counsellor friend taught me a technique which helps with panic. Breathe in to the count of seven and out to the count of eleven. The last four 'out' breaths really help to calm you down. Try to do this until the racing feeling stops. We apparently seldom exhale all the air in our lungs.

As children my mother always tried to instil in us a 'mind over matter' philosophy. Panicky screaming was completely forbidden and we had to calm ourselves in an emergency situation.

Shal was fantastic and she got me to a casualty unit in record time. My hand was swelling rapidly and somehow splinters from the pot had cut deep grooves on the top of my wrist pushing the skin back, causing it to bleed. She dropped me at the door of the hospital and went to park the car.

I was in a sort of trance as I entered the casualty department. The blood had made two perfect bracelets around my wrist and was dripping and congealing in a large blob underneath, giving the impression that my wrist had been sliced. The hand itself had swollen into a shape resembling a boxing glove. I now know this was the oedema which can accumulate at the location of a trauma and can cause serious problems with healing if it is not dispersed.

📖 For more on Oedema see pages 213 and 216

Shal joined me and in a short time I was assessed, given some painkillers and sent for an x ray. I glanced up at a poster which said "Most accidents happen in the Home".

We waited for about an hour and then I was seen by a Doctor who had viewed the x ray and was concerned.

He told us that the fracture was complicated and advised me not to eat anything as in his opinion I would probably need surgery. He explained that a Consultant had been contacted and we were asked to wait in the examination room for their arrival.

After some time another Doctor came in and asked if we wanted to see the x ray. She was curious to know how it had happened, because it was obvious that a heavy weight must have been involved. As you will see opposite, it didn't look too horrendous. I knew from the sound as the pot had crashed down onto my knuckles that there was going to be a fair amount of damage, but the visual did not seem to reflect this and so was not too shocking to me. As became obvious later though, crush injuries have their own problems.

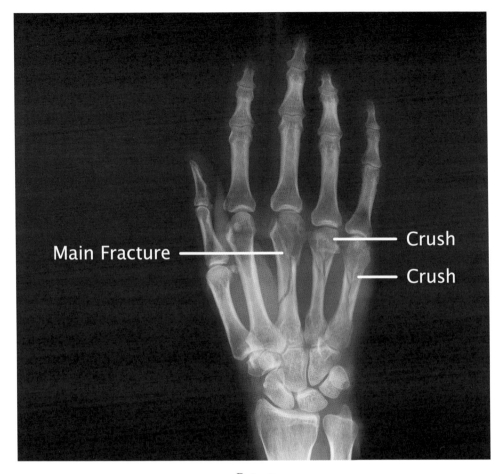

Main Fracture ——————————

Crush —————
Crush —————

Report:
There are complex intra-articular fractures of the right 3rd 4th and 5th
metacarpals at the MCP joints extending into the MCP's (big knuckles)

Eventually the original Doctor came back and said that a Consultant had looked at the x rays. Their advice was that I didn't require surgery and the cuts should be dressed and my hand and wrist set in a 'back slab'.

These are temporary casts. They consist of a half plaster cast which supports the fracture – in my case, supporting fingers, palm and wrist. A crepe bandage is then wound around the cast to hold it in place. The bandage allows for swelling and to prevent the kind of problems you can get in a full plaster. Full plasters are rigid and can restrict blood supply creating circulation problems and pain. Back slabs are pretty much standard procedure as an emergency cast and also after surgery when swelling may occur.

I was relieved that surgery had been ruled out and wanted my injury to be less serious than the doctor had first thought. So I felt quite upbeat. I was still in shock and didn't ask for a copy of the x ray at that point.

You can acquire a CD of your x ray at both NHS and private hospitals. These can cost between £10 and £30 per copy, depending on the hospital. It is useful to have a CD, but you can also request a print out, which can't be used for diagnostic purposes, but is good for keeping your own records. Ask at the reception desk when you check in for your x ray.

Two young nurses wheeled in a trolley and began preparing the plaster and chatting and giggling, which I quite liked until I noticed that one of them (who, incidentally, was not wearing surgical gloves) was wiping the blood from below my wrist, dragging the swab into the area of the cut. I pointed this out and asked her to clean the cut with alcohol. She was reticent and said that it would be extremely painful. I insisted though and said that I would prefer a quick blast of pain at that time, than an infection developing under the dressing. I was finding their banter less and less entertaining as I listened to them debate the angle the cast should be for my particular injury.

Alarm bells should have been deafening at that moment, but they weren't. I still felt too dazed. Everything is always much clearer in hindsight. If you have the slightest doubt about what is happening to you, and you have the strength to do so, question it and ask for a second opinion. This may make the person dealing with you irritable, but you are probably going to find that if you take control of your recovery, some of those treating you are going to get irritable anyway. They have so little time with each patient that one who asks questions can become an annoyance. I am not suggesting any form of abusive behaviour, only that you trust your instincts. You are the one who is going to have to live with the consequences. Those few extra minutes could mean so much to your future wellbeing. On the upside, many in the medical profession will deliver real care and will be eager to share your findings and celebrate with you when you accomplish certain goals. The open mindedness of these individuals' stems from them not having been beaten down by the system. They will want to be able to share in any new discovery that they can pass on to their other patients. Hold on to these people jealously!

Meanwhile back in the emergency room the two nurses eventually made a decision about the angle of the cast and once it was in place, they tried to put my arm in a sling. It was far too painful and sent pains shooting up from my elbow into my elevated little finger, so they gave up and explained that I would just have to hold my lower arm and hand up day and night. From now on I will refer to this as 'the wave position'.

I was told to attend the fracture clinic on the following Thursday (six days time). As we left I felt reasonably content, as psychologically and physically after having had my injury dressed, bandaged and cast, it felt clean and safe and supported. I think that at that point my body gave way to the tiredness. Shal insisted I stay the night with them so she could look after me. It had been exhausting, emotionally as well as physically. I also very quickly realised the implications of managing with one hand, while keeping the other elevated. We joked about the wave position.

Since I live on my own I really needed to assure myself that I could cope so the next morning, against Shal's wishes for me to stay, I decided to go home. I wanted to get used to the injury and work out strategies for managing the predicted six weeks in plaster. Rob, Shal's husband and my very close friend, dropped me outside the block of flats where I live and I said goodbye and managed to let myself in the front door. It was when I tried to open the door to my flat that I realised I was in trouble; the door as usual was double locked. This meant that to unlock it I had to pull the door handle towards me with one hand whilst turning the key with the other and with only one functioning hand this was now an insurmountable task. Eventually my neighbour helped me but I was left feeling frustrated and upset that this simple fracture could render me so helpless. Then I thought about all those who have lost hands in accidents or wars and received not even the most basic treatment or help from friends or neighbours and on top of all my other emotions I felt guilty and spoilt. I have to say at that moment I had no reason to doubt that I would be better soon.

By the Sunday though, I had begun to feel very afraid because the pain I was experiencing was so extreme. I had been unable to sleep and was in tears with the intensity of it. It throbbed and in spite of high doses of Ibuprofen and Paracetamol which I had been taking every four hours, I had only moments of relief. I was now feeling less brave and felt sure that there was something unusual happening in my hand. Over time though I realised how useful Ibuprofen is in relieving the effects of inflammation.

For now I decided to take myself back to the accident and emergency unit. My friend Bonita agreed to come to the hospital with me and helped me to wash and get dressed. Complicated in the wave position! I learnt very quickly that trying to wash one hand without the use of the other is a most peculiar and frustrating venture.

I discovered that it is better to use a smaller, thinner towel which can be managed easily with one hand, even after bathing. I found it much safer than a large one. Those reflexes which kicked in when I tried to control a heavy bath towel, and stop it from dropping, usually resulted in bouts of withering pain. Later I cut up one of my towels into manageable quarters and felt much more comfortable drying myself in that way.

Often it is the simplest tasks that become the most frustrating, for instance trying to put my bra on using one hand, with the other one in the wave position. I turned the bra around so that the clasps were in front and then manoeuvred it into a position that I could connect the two clasps and I would almost succeed and then it would spring open and I would try to grab it, and my reflex was to stop it with the injured elbow slamming into my waist, which was like being hit with a cricket bat. I would then be on the floor in agony for a couple of minutes and then try again. I have to say – sometimes you have to laugh otherwise you cry and in those first weeks I did manage to see the funny side in spite of the pain. Later it wasn't always so easy to laugh.

Meanwhile my left hand was having a crash course in doing things it had never done before. My right hand was experiencing a range of such excruciatingly painful sensations that I could barely think about anything else.

Bonita and I set out for the casualty department at the hospital. All the while my hand was in the wave position and throbbing. My arm was beginning to ache from holding it up. The cast felt so sickeningly tight around my swollen hand even though it was only a 'back slab'.

Bonita and I both love walking so we took advantage of the beautiful sunny day and walked all the way to the hospital. It crossed my mind at this time that I was glad that the injury had not been to my foot, which would have taken away my independence in so many more ways. The pain, by this time had completely engulfed me and I found myself caught between trying to keep my hand elevated and trying to protect it at the same time. Beneath the plaster I felt as though the skin was being stung, scorched, twisted and the flesh and bone throbbed.

When we arrived at the hospital there was a wait of about an hour. I had brought with me a large writing pad. Over the previous few days, I had been fiddling around with a pen and paper trying to write with my left hand and had begun writing about what was happening to me. It gave a purpose to the task. This in effect became the writing of a diary and recording of my injury and treatment. It was a good idea for me and taught me a lot about the relationship between my right and left hands. It also ensured that I could express, even if only to myself, the extreme pain and confusion which had suddenly arrived in my life, without losing track of the day to day.

It is a good idea to keep a diary of what is happening to you and changes that occur so you can list them to make good use of time when with your health professional. Try to do this from the beginning. I know that this sounds a bit much to ask during a traumatic time, but if you keep your own records, you can review them before appointments and it will help you to feel as though you are involved in managing your condition. In the long term it can help you to avoid repeating mistakes and should your hospital file be misplaced, you will have copies of your records. If you are on multiple medications, at least you will have notes of these, so that you will be able to record which ones really helped and which ones had side effects. If you find it difficult to write a diary as such, just keep a note each day of how your injury feels. What is your mood like? If you have had an appointment, what the doctor said, any further recommendations etc. Sometimes, even in the midst of overwhelming pain I felt confident when I went for medical appointments, because even if those treating me were unclear about what was going on I felt that I was actively involved in charting my recovery. Often you will not see the same healthcare professional you saw last time. In my case I was pleased to have a project which was so important since I was feeling isolated due to the pain. As it happened, this diary idea was good because the CRPS which was eventually diagnosed made the situation much more long term than a 'normal' fracture.

Actually it is useful to keep a record of your health in the long term anyway. You can usually get cheap page-a-day diaries at 'pound shops' which give you lots of room to write comments etc. For those who are familiar with computers you can make a table or use Excel.

📖 **For NHS advice see page 167**

Meanwhile as we waited to be seen, Bonita and I sat trying to write, me with my left because I am right handed and her with her right because she is left handed. I found it very strange to begin with and there was a resistance.

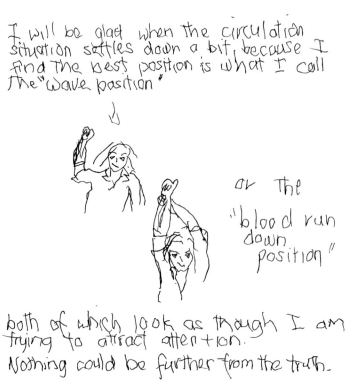

I will be glad when the circulation situation settles down a bit, because I find the best position is what I call the "wave position"

or The "blood run down position"

both of which look as though I am trying to attract attention.
Nothing could be further from the truth.

My first drawing and some writing with my left hand

Within a few days I had realised that I was expecting my left hand to deliver the same style of handwriting as the right one. Therein was the source of the resistance. As soon as I allowed it to write in its own way, it flowed much more easily. Never-the-less whenever I wrote or tried to draw with my left hand, my right hand would cramp in protest. It didn't appear to do this with other activities, like washing a cup etc. As I was to learn later, observing and making use of the relationship between both hands was not only interesting but was to prove important to my recovery.

Finally a doctor ushered us through to an examination room. She had looked at the x ray and explained that if they redid the back slab it would still just be another emergency room cast and that it was in my interests to wait for my appointment on the Thursday at the fracture clinic. She assured me that because of the nature of the injury my hand would be extremely painful and gave me some very strong pain killers and some anti-inflammatory drugs which were compatible with the painkillers. I was told not to use Ibuprofen with these particular pain killers.

Up till that point I had been taking Ibuprofen and Paracetamol four times a day which had been prescribed on the day of the accident. They are pretty much the only pain medication I ever take, and very rarely at that as I'm not keen on painkillers. I'm fearful of the long term side effects on the stomach when taking them regularly. I had one occasion to use other very strong pain-killers for a couple of weeks and the constipation which resulted was arguably more painful and frightening than the original ailment. I feel that in most cases the pain is there as a signal to guide you, to a certain extent. Not everyone would agree with me on that. This was handed down by my mother who taught us that you should listen to your body's signals and trust your immune system. She also believed and still does, that often the treatment of illness requires a certain amount of exercising mind over matter, and not rushing immediately for the pill box.

I have always agreed with her about that, but up until now, apart from a few hours when I was in labour with my son, I had never encountered either the intensity or the range of pain which was now relentlessly dogging me. I accepted the two white boxes of medication with trepidation, on the one hand, (excuse the pun) but on the other feeling that at least if the pain continued to be as shocking as it had been the night before, I had these pills which might numb me so that I could get some sleep.

Apart from the racking pain I was still very worried about the way my hand was constantly changing colour and temperature. I understood the point of having the cast changed at the fracture clinic where I hoped I could ask questions and resolved to try and hold out for the appointment. I also decided in desperation to try the stronger painkillers.

I took them for the first time that night and although they did relieve much of the pain, they were so strong that when I had to get up in the small hours I felt dizzy and had to hold onto the wall so as not to fall over. When I woke up the next day I felt sea sick and unsteady on my feet, which was very dangerous under the circumstances. The last thing I needed at that point was to fall. I didn't take them again and relied on the Ibuprofen and Paracetamol which did help to dull the pain slightly.

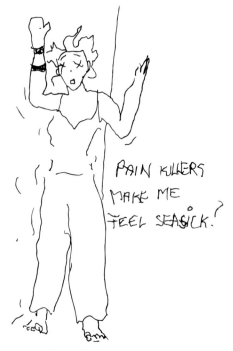

Staggering from the effects of the pain medication

Haze of Pain

By the time Thursday came I was feeling weary from lack of sleep, but never the less hopeful. My friend Elizabeth came with me to the Fracture Clinic and although my hand was very painful and bruised I was trying to be upbeat. We were laughing about the wave position and how to avoid cabs thinking that I was hailing them or shop assistants thinking I was trying to attract their attention. After the compulsory hour's wait I was sent for an x ray and then we were met by a charming doctor who, unfortunately showed scant interest in my x ray which was on the computer screen in front of him. In fact he seemed more interested in trying to guess what Elizabeth and I did for a living.

Elizabeth became irritated and said "Excuse me. I am curious. Others who have looked at this x ray expressed some alarm at the fracture and were immediately interested in how it could have happened. You seem unfazed by it and appear to feel that all is perfectly well." His reply was exactly what I wanted to hear.

"No I am not worried at all. Look." He pointed to the split down my middle metacarpal. "Look how well it has healed." This was six days after the accident and I was really pleased that the bones were healing well.

He then went on to instruct the plaster technician to fashion a fibreglass cast, cutting back the area supporting my knuckles.

I was alarmed at these instructions and having just acquired a photocopy of my x ray I showed it to the technician. He seemed as concerned as I was about the decision to remove the support to my fingers and knuckles and asked if he could take the x ray with him to discuss this with the doctor. He came back and said that the doctor knew that it was not 100% correct, but had instructed him to go ahead with cutting back the plaster. This meant that the very location of the crush injury, was receiving very little support.

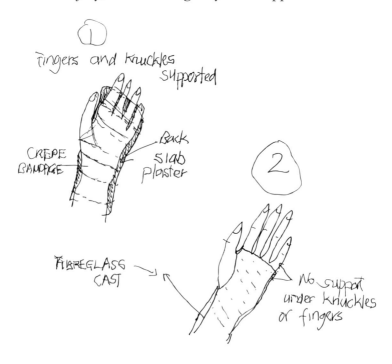

I should never have gone along with that decision. This would have been a time to have asked for a second opinion. It would probably have made me unpopular for taking up time, but I became unpopular later anyway because I was in so much pain. If that kind of decision had been made about plumbing in my flat, or the installation of an appliance, I would have challenged it without hesitation. I am always polite and realise that most of the time the lack of a good service is not the fault of the person who is sitting in front of you, so there is nothing to be gained from being aggressive. But I later wished that I had taken that step. My mother's "don't make a fuss policy" unfortunately overrode my instinct.

As is now evident, I did go along with it and Elizabeth and I chatted to the technician as he sawed away at the plaster. He told us he was ex army. We talked about how much skill doctors acquire on the frontline in a war zone and how advanced the medicines and dressings have to be because most of the time everything has to be done at such speed. I felt confident as I watched how precisely he worked. He then gave me a choice of colour of a fibreglass cast. I chose an uplifting bright green. When he had finished he still seemed unsure about the lack of support for my fingers and splinted them together with tape so that they could support each other. I later learned this was called Buddy Strapping. That technician was one of the few people I instinctively trusted during this stage of the treatment, but he was just there to fill in for someone on leave, so I never saw him again.

The fibreglass cast, unfortunately even though it had been expertly fitted, had little sharp edges around my thumb which scratched and chaffed.

Over the next few days I suffered a lot of different kinds of pain. Shooting, bruising, stinging and I noticed that my thumb and forefinger which were not fractured appeared to be bruised sometimes and then not at others. My other three fingers changed colour like cuttlefish. I found it very strange, but since I have never had a bad fracture before, I assumed this must be a 'normal' symptom. Much later I was lucky enough to attend an Occupational Therapy Unit (OT Unit) where all my questions were answered and I understood why this happens and why my uninjured finger and thumb were as painful as the injured ones.

Using diagrams, the therapist explained how the Median, Radial and Ulnar nerves *innervate* – (provide touch sensation and stimulate muscles with nerve impulses). So if there is nerve damage at the source of the injury, other locations which are innervated by that nerve will also be affected. There was obviously damage to more than one nerve at the location of my injury. I hope that the following drawings will shed some light on how it all works.

It certainly made more sense to me and I wished that I had known this right from the beginning. Having looked up pictures of nerves in the hand I felt very sure that the location of the crush must have delivered some nerve damage.

The shaded areas on the following drawings show the areas innervated by the three nerves.

Dorsal view of area innervated by the Median, Radial and Ulnar Nerves

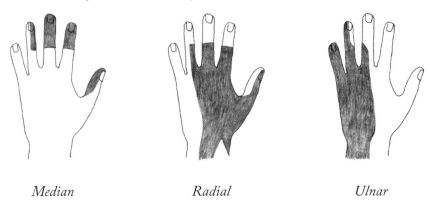

| *Median* | *Radial* | *Ulnar* |

Palmar view of area innervated by the Median, Radial and Ulnar Nerves

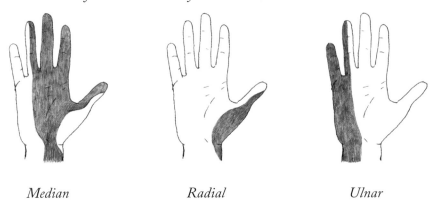

| *Median* | *Radial* | *Ulnar* |

Definitions with reference to the hand:
Dorsal – Knuckle side, Palmar – Palm side

Ask questions. It can't do any harm and sometimes you can strike it lucky and someone will take the trouble to really answer you in a way that makes your symptoms seem less of a mystery and less frightening. There is that saying that "a little knowledge can be dangerous", but being completely in the dark can be terrifying. I soon found that some healthcare professionals really appreciate feedback.

By now I was walking around in a haze of pain, trying to keep my posture correct so that my whole body didn't go into stress. I had pins and needles in my fingers and they were now trying to claw, which put an enormous pressure on the underside of my knuckles. Because the support had been removed from that area it was pure agony.

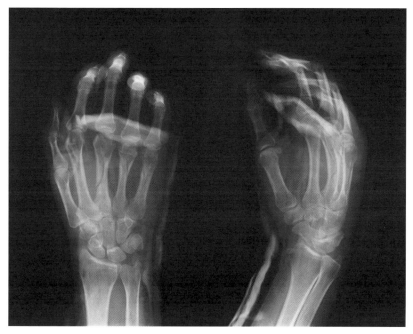

X ray of the new position of my fingers

My hand changed temperature constantly and my skin felt at one moment as though it was being singed with a blowlamp followed a few seconds later by the sensation that it had been caught in a freezing wind.

Although I was trying to 'keep my chin up' my friend Pam said that she could see the pain in my eyes. I felt grateful for that comment, because those who have experienced pain will know how lonely it is and how comforting it is when someone recognises what you are going through without dwelling on it too much. Sometimes though, I would be sitting at the table talking one moment and the next I would be on the floor in the foetal position, so the pain would be obvious. This was now day 9.

On the following pages are two illustrations showing the nerves in the hand and illustrated for me very clearly that the pains I was experiencing appeared to follow the path of the nerves. They are taken from **The Anatomy of the Human Body**, 1918. By Henry Gray (1821–1865)

Superficial Palmar nerves

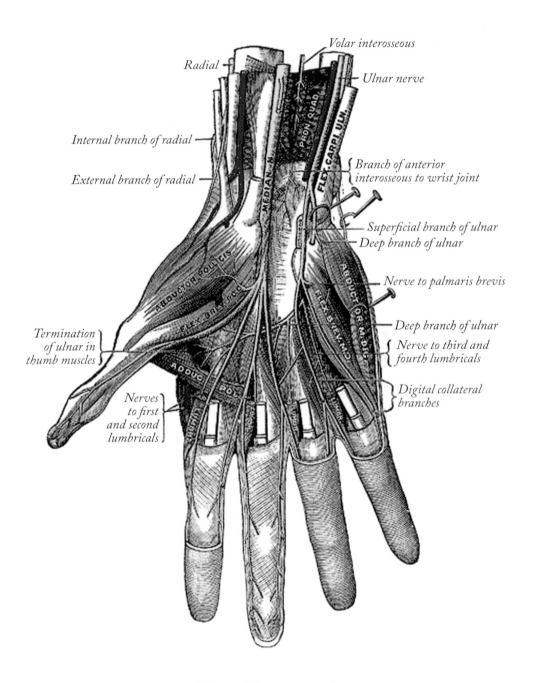

Radial

Volar interosseous

Ulnar nerve

Internal branch of radial

External branch of radial

{ Branch of anterior
  interosseous to wrist joint

Superficial branch of ulnar
Deep branch of ulnar

Nerve to palmaris brevis

Deep branch of ulnar
{ Nerve to third and
  fourth lumbricals

{ Digital collateral
  branches

Termination }
of ulnar in }
thumb muscles }

Nerves }
to first }
and second }
lumbricals }

Henry Gray 1821–1865

Deep Branch of Ulnar Nerves

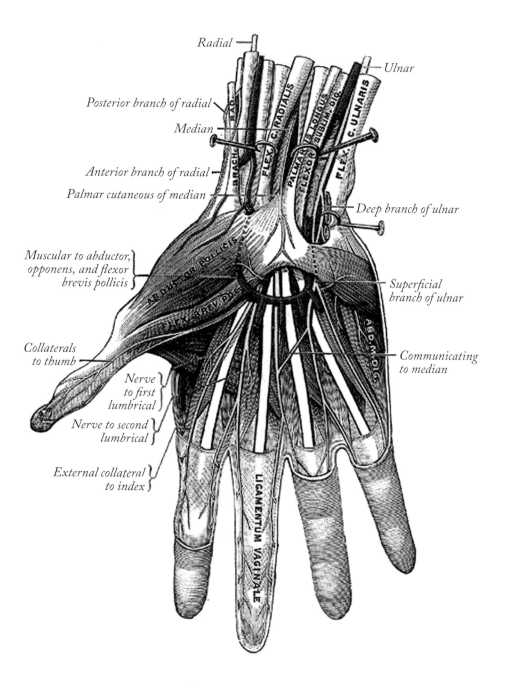

Henry Gray 1821–1865

Another friend May had been on a mission to find things to help me to cope with my present situation. She had bought me several devices designed to help someone using only one hand. First prize went to a rubber disc, looking much like a placemat, an inch or so bigger than a CD. It is a simple and ingenious method of getting tight lids off jars and bottles with one hand. All you have to do is stand the required jar etc on the ring and apply down pressure and it sticks to the rubber and you can then, while still applying down pressure, turn the lid and the jar itself does not spin or fall over. It gave me so much independence so simply. I never went anywhere without it. Thanks May.

Much later (again in the OT Unit I mentioned before) I was to discover that there are so many products which are fantastically helpful for anyone managing either with only one hand or indeed any condition which imposes limitations on daily activities. I was shown a catalogue which was a revelation in ways to maintain independence. Independence in itself creates a degree of movement and activity, all of which are very important for recovery. Some of the items may be expensive, but even if you can manage just one item that will help you, it really is worth it. Below is a round anchor pad (rubber disc as mentioned above) and jar opener.

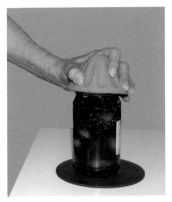
Round anchor pad and jar opener

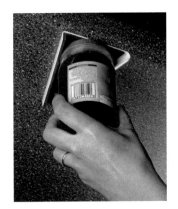
Undo-it jar and bottle opener

📖 **For contact and catalogue information see Patterson / Homecraft on page 239**

May had understood very quickly how difficult one handedness was going to be. Every day the frustration list was growing. Trying to get a toothbrush out of its high security packaging, for instance, had always been a problem, it was now completely impossible. Everything these days seems to be cling wrapped and sealed so tightly that you can actually damage yourself or the product trying to get it out of the packaging! A lot of new products including some foodstuffs had become completely out of my reach. I could see them languishing within their stout packaging, but all I could do was imagine what it would be like to have access to them.

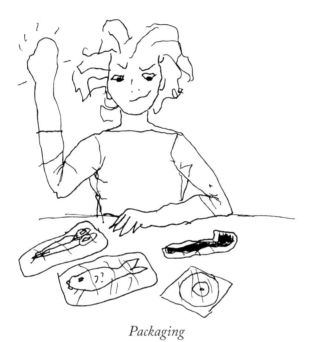

Packaging

Over the next week, my hand continued to feel alternatively as though scalded with boiling water or frostbitten and I had begun to feel quite sorry for myself. I was trying to put on a brave face, but this was becoming increasingly difficult as my upper body was beginning to contort with the pain. I also realised that although I wanted to convince others and myself that I was coping, doing that, in itself can become isolating. Two weeks of relentless pain can seem like a very long time and it can make you feel completely outside of normal life. Experiencing constant pain is like having a loud incessant noise in your body that no-one else can hear.

At this time three of my close friends were bravely fighting cancer and undergoing extremely unpleasant treatments with the minimum of fuss. I just had a broken hand! I felt really embarrassed about what was happening to me and so tried to play down just how devastating the pain was. Everyone around me was always so happy to hear that I was feeling better, that I felt as though I didn't want to disappoint them. However, the searing waves of pain I was now encountering were so violent that at times I did find them difficult to conceal. Those in pain will know, it is at night, when you are kept awake wondering what is going on under your skin to cause such exaggerated sensations, when you yearn for sleep, that you begin to feel afraid and very alone.

It was also around this time that I realised that I had injured both knees when I tripped getting out of the car, on the day of the accident. I was at Rob and Shal's house and Rob was sitting on the couch. As I was leaving, I bent down to kiss him goodbye and our knees touched and I screamed in agony (so much for Ms Cool!) I felt like I had just been hit with a crowbar, a hot, violent pain. I took myself off to my local GP surgery and was seen by a very empathetic doctor who explained that there was an accumulation of fluid on my knees and that the best thing I could do to relieve this was to push icy compresses as hard as I could against them. She warned that this would incur 'some discomfort', but that it would help bring down the inflammation.
I liked her a lot. Sadly that was the last time I saw her as she went on maternity leave for a year. The second person I trusted – gone!
'Some discomfort' was a little understated. I felt like I was pushing a red hot poker against my knees and there was a strange 'creak' and then the fluid seemed to retreat away from the compress like some jellyfish fleeing from danger. It had the desired effect though and brought down the inflammation. My knees still felt sensitive a year later and kneeling was pretty impossible. I have to be emphatic here:

> *Do not do anything like this*
> *without consulting a professional first!*
> *This is a record of how I coped with my injuries,*
> *but I always consulted health professionals.*
>
> *What worked for me may not be right for you!*

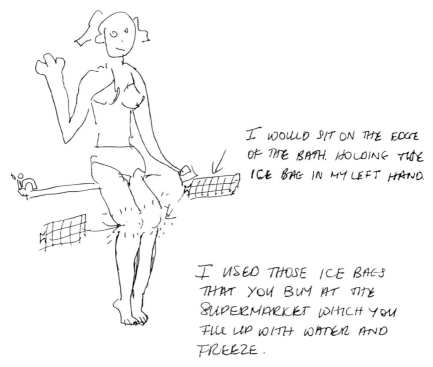

I WOULD SIT ON THE EDGE OF THE BATH. HOLDING THE ICE BAG IN MY LEFT HAND.

I USED THOSE ICE BAGS THAT YOU BUY AT THE SUPERMARKET WHICH YOU FILL UP WITH WATER AND FREEZE.

Taking care of my knees

By this time my whole right arm had become racked with pain and I was conscious that I could easily knock it and so tried to protect it at all times, which is difficult when you are in the wave position.

I sleep alone in a double bed pushed against the wall in the corner of the room. Because of the requirement of the wave position, I had found a way to prop myself up into the corner and pile pillows and cushions around my arm, to take some of the strain out of constantly holding it up in the air.

Now! With my knees in pain and my right arm in the wave position, getting onto the bed and into the corner left me the limiting option of flopping down like a seal and manoeuvring myself in that way into position. The down side of this was that my pyjama top would invariably become twisted around my neck or I would lose the bottoms. Re-arranging them was infuriating and frustrating. Getting up in the night was a major production.

On a more serious note, if I accidentally fell onto the injured arm or hand I would be racked with indescribable pain. Trust me this happened often.

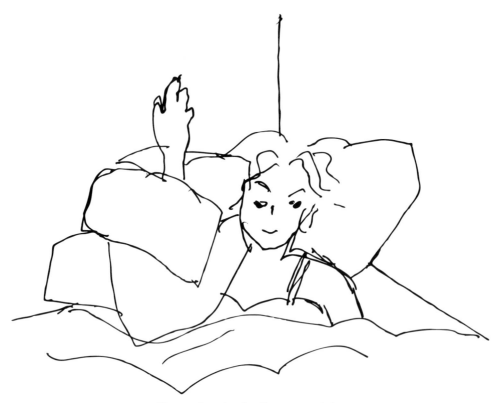

Propped up in the Corner at night.

Much, much later I discovered the V shaped support pillow. It weighs significantly less than most others and whereas I had to try to control a set of pillows
to support my shoulder and hand, this one pillow could do the job. It certainly
would have been a lot easier to handle in the early stages and I am sure would
have been a lot more therapeutic for my shoulder which was doing all the work
in keeping my hand elevated. I later also realised that for someone dealing
with injuries to both hands these are indispensible and because of the shape
and weight, they can easily be lifted by resting in the cusp of the elbow. Try
using two. Friends who I had told about the V Pillow have reported that they
are as effective in elevating legs and for using as support for the back and neck.

It may be that the very act of keeping the wave position was adding to the
problem, but it was most certainly the least painful option at that time.

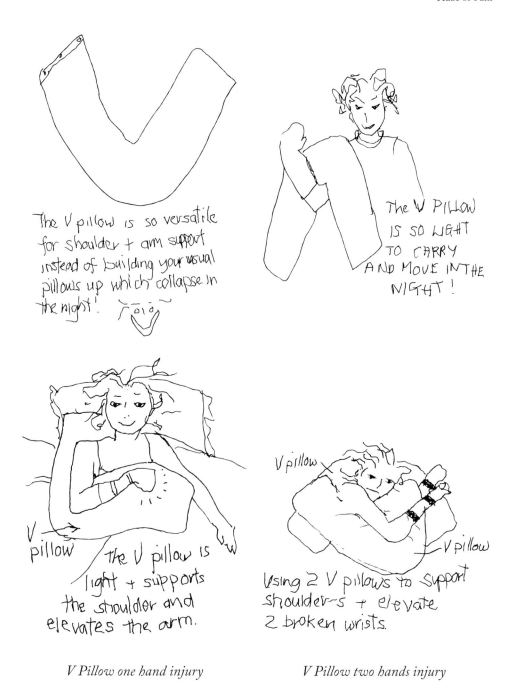

The V pillow is so versatile for shoulder + arm support instead of building your usual pillows up which collapse in the night!

The V PILLOW IS SO LIGHT TO CARRY AND MOVE IN THE NIGHT!

V pillow   The V pillow is light + supports the shoulder and elevates the arm.

V pillow   V pillow   Using 2 V pillows to support shoulders + elevate 2 broken wrists.

V Pillow one hand injury

V Pillow two hands injury

📖 **These V Shaped Pillows are available from Argos see page 239**

On the Thursday I went to my appointment at the fracture clinic and was seen by yet another doctor and when he saw my hand he was immediately concerned at the lack of support to my fingers and gave instructions for the cast to be removed and another one made to support them entirely. I felt quite relieved and was duly fitted with the next cast although I was slightly worried that this was the third time my hand had been set. The technician was really careful not to move it too much as he installed the latest cast. Now you could barely see the tips of my fingers.

The unit was so busy. It was like a factory conveyor belt and most of the practitioners looked exhausted. I imagine it is difficult for the doctors and other health workers to pay the sort of attention to their patients that they might like to.

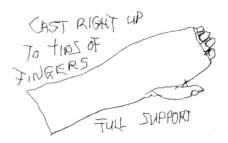

Well, so there I was on day 14 and in my third cast. I liked the doctor I saw this time and he explained that it was a complicated injury and made a note to refer me for Occupational Therapy. This referral was one of the few really positive aspects of those early days.

He then prescribed an anti-biotic for the cuts which were under the dressing as a preventative measure and asked me to make an appointment to come back to the fracture clinic after two weeks. I made a note of his name. I felt safe with him.

Always make a note of the name of the person who has treated you. I think it is important for the doctor patient relationship. Apart from that, it is quite important to keep clear records. I know that there is a growing litigious population in this country. Following the American Model, there are ambulance chasers and many others who would like to make a quick buck out of the system. This can make some in the medical profession very uneasy if you attempt to keep your own records. Don't let this deter you, you are entitled to your records and not all of us who do so are seeking to find evidence for law suits or to 'make trouble'.

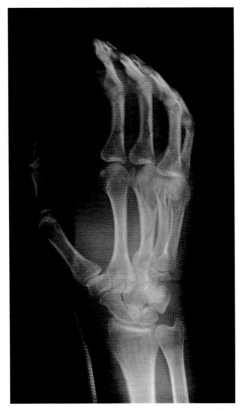

The new cast was supporting my knuckles.

📖 **For advice on how to access NHS health records see page 167**

Meanwhile, I had been working on eating with chopsticks using my left hand and was becoming quite adept at it.

I found that using a fork in that hand, without a knife was a disaster. Food kept flying off the plate. I was a one woman demolition crew. Clumsy eating was a not a look that I wanted to develop. However! Chopsticks gave me more control because of the pincer movement.

On the Saturday May invited me over for a meal with Pam and Victor and some friends. The food, as always with May, was delicious.

I am proud to announce that I was able to eat everything, including some sorbet, using chopsticks and in the wave position.

I didn't stay long at May's after eating, because my hand had now developed a whole new range of painful sensations. The palm felt as though it was being sanded raw with a rough grade of sandpaper. The fingers felt as though they were twisted around each other while someone wrung them like a wet towel. My cuticles felt as though they were being pushed back harshly as if my hand was being drawn into a tight tube too narrow for it, and yet, if you looked at the tips of my fingers, which were barely visible, they looked fine and pink and healthy. I was also encountering cramps and shooting pains up and down my arm which was constantly changing temperature.

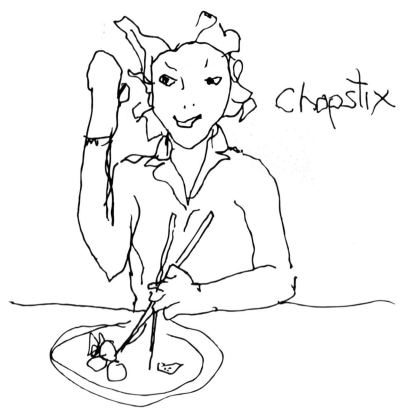

Chopsticks were a solution to the eating problem

This is a time when I did a lot of weeping with the pain. I was very afraid when I was on the underground or in the street that someone might bump into me and jar my arm. The positive feeling I had in the beginning that it would all be over soon was replaced by a deep concern and quite frankly – fear. I couldn't believe that the pain I was experiencing was a healing pain. It was too restricting, too crushing.

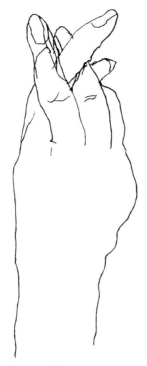

My fingers felt twisted in a cramp

Later in the year I was prompted by a friend to speak to Demian, a friend of hers who had lost one eye and one hand in an accident. He became an inspiration to me, not only because of his enthusiasm for passing on findings that had been useful to him, but he understood the pain I was experiencing. I am jumping ahead here, but anyone experiencing CRPS will understand how difficult it is to acquire this kind of information, so I'm not going to delay for the sake of chronology. Demian helped me to understand that the symptoms I was experiencing were almost certainly the result of nerve damage. When I described the twisted and the tugging feelings in my hand and wrist, he recognised them immediately and said that he had experienced exactly the same sensations in his 'phantom hand'. He told me that in the beginning he sometimes felt as though he was making such a tight fist that he could feel his phantom fingernails biting into his palm in spite of the physical absence of that hand.

📖 **For more on Phantom Limb Pain see page 185**

He made me realise that there was a connection between my pain and that experienced by an amputee. He explained that it was extremely likely that when the pot crashed down it did some damage to one or more nerves in my hand. Due to the trauma they had begun sending confused messages to the brain, creating this range of excruciating symptoms. It was exactly what I had supposed was happening having studied many anatomical drawings. Demian is also very upbeat in the way he approaches the physical losses that he has experienced. He, like me, made a very early decision to avoid becoming addicted to pain killers. A very brave choice in his case! Demian's accident happened over 20 years ago in South America. He had been at a party and he was sitting beside a glass table near the pool, when a firework landed on the table and exploded the glass in great shards in every direction. His hand and eye were irreversibly damaged and a substantial area around his temple lacerated. His hand was amputated and several surgical procedures were performed on his temple.

Demian decided to seek out complementary medicine or alternatives to conventional medicine during his recovery. Later this decision was compounded when back in Germany he had to attend a hospital for some treatment and found many war veterans with amputations and severely painful injures simply languishing in units where they were delivered massive doses of morphine and other highly addictive medications for the pain and little else. Of course Demian applauds the surgery which saved his life and some of the various main stream treatments, but on the whole he was more impressed by the alternative and complimentary therapies he used over the years because of the lack of side effects.

I'll return to the support that Demian gave me later, but in the meantime I need to go back to the Monday (four days after) my attendance at the fracture clinic where a cast had been applied for the third time.

ALEXANDER TECHNIQUE AND FRACTURE CLINIC

I was now worried that my posture was suffering from the strange way I had to hold my arm and the position that I was forced to adopt when sleeping. From time to time I attempted to use a sling to give some rest to my shoulder but in every case electrifying pains would shoot from my elbow into my little finger and so I would have to abandon that idea. I had to keep my hand elevated because if I didn't it throbbed and ached even more dramatically than it did when in the 'wave position'. It also very quickly became more swollen. Now my shoulder ached constantly and my back felt tender and vulnerable, often an indication that something was going to go wrong with it, which is the last thing I needed at that stage. I knew that it was early days as far as my fracture was concerned, but the obvious effect on the rest of my body also needed to be addressed.

I have always been interested in therapies where success depends on the participation of the patient. I think that psychologically it is helpful to feel as though you are working at recovery, particularly where chronic pain symptoms leave you feeling helpless. I had a fall as a child and slipped a disc in my lower back. In my latter years it began to be a nuisance and a friend had introduced me to The Alexander Technique. It is an extremely quiet and gentle treatment. It teaches you to become very aware of your posture and helps you to align your spine, keep any strain off your neck and make good use of breathing. The practitioners call themselves teachers, which I like, because it implies that they are going to impart their knowledge, teach you how to maintain good posture, among many other things, so that you have input and can work at The Technique on your own.

📖 **For details on The Society of Teachers of the Alexander Technique (STAT) see page 199**

📖 **For the origins and history of the Alexander Technique see page 229**

Anyway on that Monday I went to see Lizzy who had been my Alexander teacher for 12 years. Usually I would only go to see her when my back became a problem. This was probably once a year or so if I had lifted something heavy or been sitting badly in front of the computer. Lizzie always encouraged me to repeat the subtle techniques which she taught me, as many times during my day as possible. I have to say in my experience it makes an enormous difference. Alexander Technique is known to be very effective in managing back pain, among many other painful conditions. Actually sometimes the effectiveness of something like Alexander is so quick that the amount of time spent in pain is reduced radically. You can practise the technique at home. It is really useful if you strain yourself or wake up with a stiff neck etc.
The relief it gives helps to sustain movement and prevent unwanted awkward posture which is so important.

On this particular morning Lizzie very gently tried to help me to concentrate on relaxing my neck, but by now I was in such stress that I was afraid of anyone touching me and had become very protective of my arm so I couldn't relax. I was pretty much in tears as the waves of pain swept up and down my arm. Lizzie, who often works with clients who use Acupuncture, suggested very wisely that perhaps Acupuncture would be a better option for me at that point because of the swelling and I could come back to Alexander later. (Alexander Technique and Acupuncture complement each other) I had had Acupuncture once for stress during bereavement, so I knew what it was about. Although I trusted Lizzy's opinion implicitly on these matters, the idea of having someone put needles anywhere near my arm or hand made me wince.

A new pain had arrived on the scene. It felt like a sharp blow with a small hammer on the nail of my middle finger. I would feel the 'blow' and then a couple of seconds later a tsunami of pain would travel along the edges of that finger, through my hand, proceed up my arm, electrify my elbow and then sweep on up to my shoulder where it felt as though I was being stabbed and then it dissipated as sharply as it had begun.

My thumb was sometimes black and blue and at other times a strange grey colour. My elbow was the colour of a pale aubergine, as though I had dipped it deeply into a pot of ink. I wept with pain as I sat talking to Lizzie on the treatment bed. I was sure the cast was wrong. Lizzie said I should trust my judgement and go back to the hospital if I thought there was something amiss. I did return to Alexander later but for the moment I took Lizzie's advice about trusting my judgement and went off back to the hospital where although it wasn't a fracture clinic day I managed to have an x ray done.

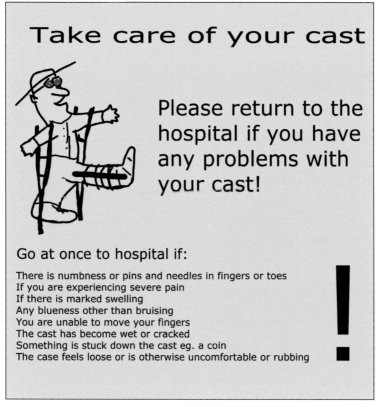

Pamphlet similar to the one from the Fracture Clinic

It apparently showed no irregularities, although I was not actually shown the results. This didn't in any way make me feel less worried and I had the added concern that due to building maintenance work at the clinic I would not have another appointment for three weeks instead of two.

I was terrified of being left on my own with the pain for that amount of time and clutching a little pamphlet that had been given to me on that first day in casualty I resolved to turn up at the Thursday fracture clinic (in two days time) even though I didn't have an appointment.

At this point, I allowed myself to think the worst. Recognising that the pain I was enduring could not possibly be normal, I began to believe that maybe there was something terribly wrong and that nobody was noticing and my hand was in serious danger and I had to remain very pro-active. People kept saying "Don't worry, fractures take time to heal." "You have had a bad fracture. It is going to be very painful, but you really must take strong painkillers all the time. They will make you feel better!" I kept thinking back over all the people I had ever seen in casts and wondered if they had all been in the kind of pain I was now experiencing.

"I don't believe any of them. I'm scared!"

Excerpt from my diary.

Saved

My friend Mimi came over to stay the night with me, which I was quite pleased about as I was feeling very vulnerable. During the night I got up and when I was getting back into bed, I slipped and brushed against the wall which delivered an indescribable pain to my elbow and hand and for the first time since the accident, I really cried. I had wept about the pain, but now I really cried for myself, for the frustration I was feeling and for my poor hand which was suffering so much. Mimi held me gently and I realised how beneficial human touch can be when you are racked with constant pain.

That cry was so important. If you are like me and try to put on a brave face, there is a fine line between that and denying yourself the appropriate emotional outlets. I cried like a baby then and I felt a real release afterwards. For others to be held by someone may be unthinkable because of the level of pain. For me at that time it <u>was</u> valuable. It is surprising how short a time it takes for constant pain to have a psychological and emotional effect.

The next day my cousin Barbara arrived to stay with me for a few weeks in between jobs. She works as a carer for elderly people and often those with Alzheimer's or Dementia. I mention what she does because I was so fortunate to have her with me as she has a gentle but firm approach having been brought up with the same kinds of attitudes as my mother's. Apart from that, in her job she is always in contact with those who are frail, so I appreciated her quiet confidence. She cooked up soups for me which she packaged and put in the freezer and helped me with domestic stuff which had been pretty neglected. By the morning of my gate crashing of the fracture clinic, I was aware that on top of everything else, if I sniffed the tips of my fingers, there was a sour unpleasant smell coming from within the cast. Barbara made me breakfast and I left home very early and was at the hospital by 9 AM.

Once there, I found out that the fracture clinic only began at 1.30 but I saw the plaster technician who had made my last cast and told him of my concerns and he called upstairs and spoke to the doctor who I had seen on the previous appointment. He agreed to see me that afternoon during fracture clinic hours. Although this meant prolonging the agony, I went away and killed time until 1.15 PM and arrived back at the same time as the doctor.

We spoke briefly and he looked at my hand, told me that there was usually a faint smell in a cast and asked me when I had had my last x ray. I explained that I had been there on the Monday (3 days before) and was told that all was fine. I tried to describe the extreme twisting and burning sensations I was experiencing. He inspected my fingers and told me that it all looked absolutely fine and that my fingertips were pink and so it was all healthy, but if I was willing to have a long wait he would try to see me. Although I was still taking 500 mg of Ibuprofen and 500 mg of Paracetamol four times a day the pain was so severe at this stage that tears were running down my face.

The unit was beginning to fill up and I was sitting with others who were there to have plasters changed or removed and it became obvious from the conversations that were going on that the setting of fractures is not an exact science. One woman who was there with her daughter asked me "How long have you been in that cast dear?" when I told her this was my third in as many weeks, she said calmly "Yes my daughter" she indicated a young woman of about twenty two with her entire leg in a cast "Has had many casts and now she has just had her third operation." Others in the line joined in the banter about the inevitability of ongoing problems. I was really struggling with containing the pain and all this was making me feel very, very queasy. I also felt like a bit of a drama queen, with just a fractured hand when all the others in the queue had much more serious injuries. None of them seemed to be experiencing withering levels of pain. I couldn't believe it was because they were all plied full of painkillers.

It was now coming up for 3.30 and I was in such agony that I was considering phoning around to find a friend who would be willing to help me cut the cast off. I know it sounds mad, but I was panicking and it felt as though there was some restriction in the palm of my hand and a feeling of unbelievable pressure under the cast. I also had the distinct feeling from the attitude of the doctor that I was waiting to see that he considered my behaviour and description of the pain as an over-reaction. To be fair, the whole department was rushed off its feet. What worried me was that I would be seen last and the cast would remain on and I would have to go home without any relief. I felt very frightened and acutely aware that I was just one of thousands who pass through that unit every year, so although I felt as though the pain was so huge that I must surely be radiating a glow, actually I looked no different to anyone else and was just a number waiting to be called. Compared to some of the injuries which are likely to be seen there, mine was probably deemed to be relatively minor and I can fully understand that.

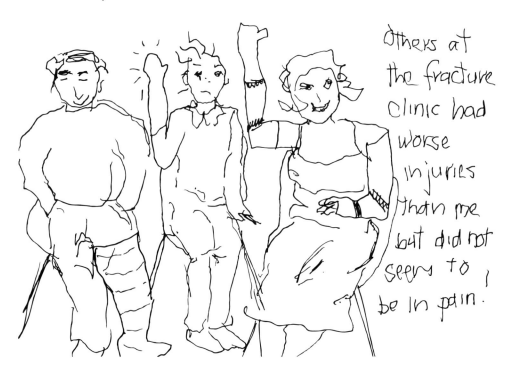

Others at the fracture clinic had worse injuries than me but did not seem to be in pain.

I felt like a Prima Donna

In retrospect I realised that if there had been more awareness at every level about CRPS, the array of disproportionate pains would have been read as a clear signal of this condition and a perhaps a more careful psychological approach might have been in place very early on. Just the acknowledgement that the pain might have been CRPS would have made such a difference and made me feel less insane and isolated.

For Pain Relief Foundation see page 191 and beginning of book

Meanwhile back in the queue at the fracture clinic the idea of removing the cast myself was looking more and more attractive. I was anxious and frightened and felt very alone. The pain was enveloping me.

Shal had left for France a couple of days after my accident. I called her number to see if she was back. Thankfully she was and was horrified to hear what was happening and told me to jump in a cab and come straight over. She would in the meantime contact her private GP and ask him to come to the house.

I grabbed my trusty file which at that stage only contained 3 x rays and my diary, and informed the duty nurse that I was in so much pain, I could no longer just sit there waiting, and I caught a taxi to Shal's house.

From there on I was taken seriously and treated as though I was entitled to an opinion and that it mattered. Shal's GP looked at my x ray, smelt what could be seen of the ends of my fingers and agreed there was a sour smell and after asking me details of what had happened, got straight on the phone and by 5 PM Shal and I were sitting in front of a Consultant at a private hospital. She had waited for me to arrive from across town.

I explained briefly what I had been going through. The Consultant called in an Occupational Hand Therapist who cut the plaster off my hand. **It stank!** And it was a strange khaki colour, but the area which had been so painful, the centre of the palm, was grey and smelly. The feeling of relief was intense and I realised that my thumb had been in a strange position. Not that it would have shown on the x ray probably but I could feel the release when the plaster came off.

Shal and I went off to the x ray department and the staff there seemed very shocked at the sight of my hand. For my part, I was just so relieved at having had the cast removed. The pressure was somewhat relieved, although it was still excruciatingly painful and even trying to lay it flat on the x ray table was agony.

The consultant looked at the x ray and told me that it appeared that the fracture was holding together, but that because of the nature of the crush injury, I would lose the 'cascade' of the knuckles on that hand.

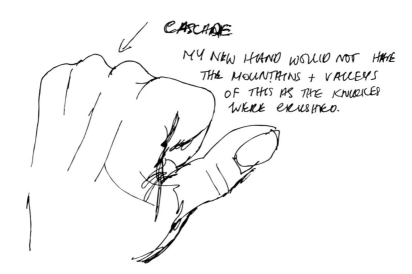

She told me that she was going to ask the Hand Therapist to make a thermoplastic splint for me and that she would like to see me the following day.

Shal insisted on paying for any treatments that I needed. This was a really important gesture, as private medicine is so expensive, and by now I knew there was an extreme urgency about treating my hand and that delays – such as had been occurring before, could be really devastating in the long term for its recovery.

The Hand Therapist (Terry) was a real perfectionist in her design of the splint. I watched as she drew a template on a piece of paper towel and then traced it onto the plastic. I was amazed at how useful the thermoplastic was. It is just a plastic sheet about a half a centimeter thick. She then cut the shape out of the plastic and lowered it into hot water with tongs. This made the plastic pliable, so that it could be moulded around my hand. Anyone who has attended a Hand Therapy unit will be familiar with these splints.

Although I was trembling with pain as she drew a tubular bandage (*compression bandage*) over my hand, with a hole cut for the thumb, I felt so confident that I was in good hands. **Literally!** She explained everything she was doing and that the Velcro straps were there so that I could take the splint off to wash and air my hand as the grey smelly area was worrying. My cousin Barbara, who helped me during the ensuing weeks to remove the cast and wash my hand, told me recently that she can still vividly recall the fetid smell emanating from my palm.

Terry stretched back the thermoplastic cast and held it open as I manoeuvred a very painful hand into position. I was quaking with fear imagining the pain if she accidentally slipped and it clicked closed in the wrong position. Of course nothing like that happened, but the fear was there. The hand was very swollen and the feel of the Velcro straps was another source of discomfort, although Terry had designed it very carefully to eliminate as much pain as possible.

She advised me for the time being to keep it elevated, as much as I could and said she would also see me the following day.

I phoned the fracture unit to cancel the appointment that I had in two weeks time. There were notices up in the hospital about this. They remind you to cancel appointments you don't need, so others can take your place. I read in a Patients Association newsletter that 6.5 million Hospital appointments were missed between 2007 and 2008, at an average cost of £100 each. That's a lot of money that could be spent on treatments. If you don't attend an appointment and don't cancel the unit will probably discharge you back to your GP anyway and you'll have to begin the whole process all over again.

📖 **For Patients Association see page 209**

Occupational Therapy and Hand Unit

"Occupational Therapy is a new healing method which is working such miracles with the mentally disordered and the victims of long and tedious convalescence."

Elizabeth Casson
Founder of the first School of Occupational Therapy in the UK 1929

From this point on I began an intensive programme of Hand Therapy – twice a week. I was filled with dread as Terry who had designed my splint explained to me that it was crucial that I got my hand moving. It was so swollen and rigid and the longer it remained that way the less likely it would be to regain movement later. The skin on my hand was now thin and shiny and felt as though it was on fire and just pulling the tubular bandage on and off was like pushing it against an emery wheel. The pain was completely out of proportion to the way people were describing fracture pains to me. The colour and temperature was changing all the time and the shooting pains, muscle contractions, stabbing sensations and cramps, which had begun over the last weeks, were now coming on fast and strong.

The hole cut in the tubular bandage for my thumb began to chafe the area between my thumb and index finger and added to the litany of painful sensations. Toni gave me an oedema glove to wear within the thermoplastic splint which would also serve to keep the swelling down. Actually from then on I used oedema gloves to keep the swelling in check. They really are fantastic and you can get them both with full finger and half finger designs. Your Hand Therapy unit will usually supply these.

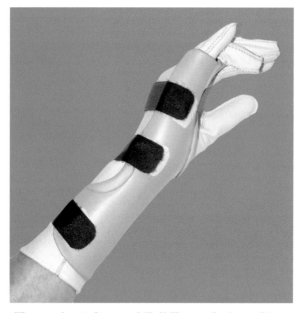

Thermoplastic Cast and Full Finger Oedema Glove

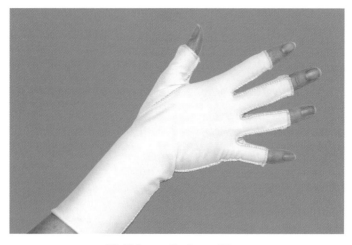

Half finger Oedema Glove

When I asked Terry how long she thought it would be before I was better, she answered that we should aim for significant improvement by Christmas (four and half months later) and complete recovery in a year. I was quite shocked that she thought it would take so long, but was determined to better the prediction date.

Around this time I received notification of my appointment at an NHS Occupational Therapy Department. This was the appointment arranged by the doctor in the fracture clinic. Although I was attending the private clinic for Hand Therapy I wanted to take up the appointment as I understood this was a long term situation and I couldn't expect my friends to continue to sponsor private treatment indefinitely.

I, like the majority of the population, have no health insurance.

Occupational Therapists are trained to work in a variety of physical and mental health settings and then often specialise in a particular area. The Occupational Therapists described in this book have specialised in Hand Therapy, but due to the profession's ethos, still try to approach patients from a perspective of the person as a whole, their life and their needs. I really recommend anyone who is suffering painful conditions to ask for a referral to an Occupational Therapy Unit. You can do this through your GP.

📖 **For The College of Occupational Therapists see page 194**

📖 **For Occupational Therapy's historical references see page 226**

On the morning of the NHS Occupational Therapy appointment I had got up at 5:30 after a painful and sleepless night and my appointment was at 9 AM. I have to say I was in so much pain that day that I don't remember much other than the sensation of walking into the Unit and immediately feeling as if I had arrived at an oasis of care. The receptionists greeted me in such a cheerful way that it lifted my spirits. Joseph the OT (Occupational Therapist) was empathic and gentle and responded carefully and thoughtfully to my questions. We decided that since I was being seen for the time being privately, I should ask for a referral back to OT later through the fracture unit. Joseph said that when I did make the appointment he would like to be present, because he wanted to discuss my hand with the consultant. I felt less frightened after that appointment because I realised that although it was obvious my condition was not short term, I had been referred to an NHS unit where I felt that there was an ethos conducive to the healing process, both physical and psychological. As I left there I felt grateful for that stroke of luck and thought about what it must be like to be suffering this kind of pain in other parts of the world without any medical support or health care of any kind and how lucky we are to have a Health Service. Without the support, I tried to imagine what strategies people develop to prevent themselves slipping into dark depression.

I continued the twice weekly Hand Therapy sessions with Terry, who is very experienced and has worked in Occupational Therapy departments in New Zealand and Australia and is very familiar with crush injuries of every nature. I asked her about the sort of injuries she had treated and she said that most crush injuries like mine occur in manufacturing situations. One patient had seen a screw below where a piston of some sort was about to come down and had tried to beat the piston and brush the screw out of the way. These kinds of injuries were quite common. She said people often had tendon injuries to their wrists after cutting open an avocado or slicing fruit with the knife cutting towards the wrist. I later met someone who had cut tendons on a sharp vegetable knife, blade pointing up in a drying rack.

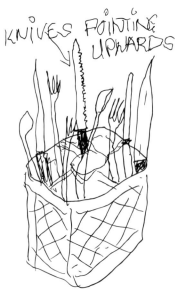

Dangerous stacking of knives

At this point my hand was rigid and incapable of any movement. Terry was strict and encouraged me to push myself to get my fingers moving. I was often in tears during the sessions, but really glad that I was able to have them and that I was not still sitting somewhere trapped in a fibreglass cast. I was also lucky to be receiving Terry's 'tough love' in Hand Therapy because it eventually helped create some movement in my hand and encouraged me to build on that movement, no matter how tiny, and not give up.

If you are taking pain medication please try to use the respite it gives you to move as much as possible and to use your limb! The Hand Therapists can show you the methods for recovery but it is up to you to keep up the exercises they give you.

Terry insisted that I spend less and less time in the splint, but advised me to sleep in it to protect my hand in case I rolled over onto it in the middle of the night. Having the splint off for periods of time during the day meant that I found myself trying to move my fingers and wrist, which was still pretty im-possible because there was still a lot of oedema and pain. I trusted her though and kept trying and eventually it paid off.

One of the exercises which I found particularly excruciating was to try to stretch my fingers apart, because it produced the most vulnerable feelings in my knuckles. It felt as though they were going to break away from each other and the pain was indescribable. I need to point out that at this stage the three injured fingers were rigidly stuck together. The only way I could dry between them when I washed was to thread the edge of a handkerchief between each one and dry them in that way. They were as stiff as boards.

Terry made me a 'Chip bag'. This is a length of tubular bandage sown up on one end into which she stuffed chopped up pieces of foam and neoprene and then sewed up the other end, joining it up like a donut. This is particularly helpful in an injury like mine to the knuckles.

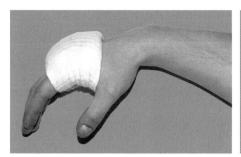 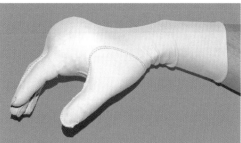

Now the idea of this is that you push your hand through the chip bag (donut) until it forms a protective buffer over the knuckles and then pull the oedema glove over the whole thing to keep it in place. Of course as anyone experiencing the kind of pain I have been describing will know, just the notion of this action is enough to make you scream out loud.

However Terry, much like my mother was not about to tolerate a wimp and to her credit (again) this device made me feel so much more secure with my knuckles cushioned from potential knocks. I could also attempt to spread my fingers sideways as the chip bag supported the knuckles. It was not painless, but it felt more like trying to move badly bruised fingers and less like they were about to snap apart.

Hand Exercises in 'Chip Bag'

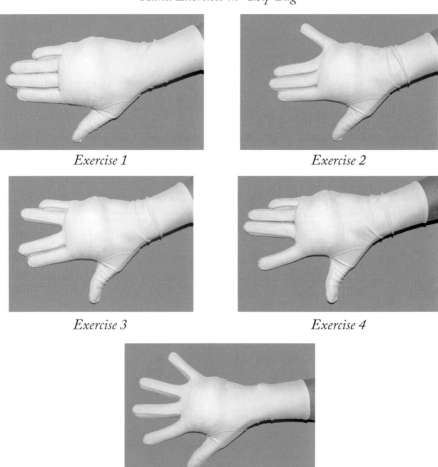

Exercise 1   *Exercise 2*

Exercise 3   *Exercise 4*

Exercise 5

Of course the full range of movements pictured were not remotely possible at all in the early stages, but were the ones that I tried to achieve.

Set yourself targets!

The 'glove and chip bag look' was quite strange as you will see from the photos opposite. Often neighbours would see me and ask how I was and look with anxiety at the shape of my hand with the chip bag under the glove. Small children would point at it with fear in their eyes.

Later when I wasn't wearing the splints anymore, the chip bag proved majorly helpful when travelling on public transport or moving in crowds. The cushioning effect it gave made it easier for me to try and avoid the protective stance of pulling my hand in close to the centre of my ribs and turning it so that it succumbed to the claw position. At this stage there was also a constant tugging sensation as though all the muscles and tendons in the arm were shrinking, involuntarily drawing my elbow in and my hand inward and upward. This stance also produced ugly cramps in the immobilised elbow.

I decided that I shouldn't look at my hand with horror and treat it as though it was an abomination. Instead I took the decision to give it praise when it achieved any movement. Instead of noting its limitations I celebrated its achievements no matter how miniscule they were. Although the extreme pain can naturally isolate an injured limb and create a tendency to protect it with strange postures, I found excluding it and treating it as though it was separate from the rest of me was a very negative approach. I worked hard on trying to feel the whole flow of my system coming to and leaving the injured hand. Now I know this may sound a little 'New Agey' for some, but it actually works. Your mind is a powerful driving force and if you engage with its power it can really help you to recover and your body is after all one system.

I believe that all of these things helped to begin the process of desensitising my skin from those acute burning and freezing sensations. These sensations stayed with me for a long time, but I realise that those early attempts to move and desensitise my skin were very important to my eventual recovery.

At this time I also became aware of the difference between active and passive movements. Passive movements are, for example, when your Hand Therapist pushes at your fingers or wrist to produce some movement which is otherwise impossible. Active movements are the ones which occur without any outside force being applied. In other words the active movement is a more natural, movement occurring because the finger or wrist is attempting to engage, or is engaging in, normal function without this outside intervention. These are the hardest movements to achieve and involve a lot of concentration to overcome the notion of "I can't"!

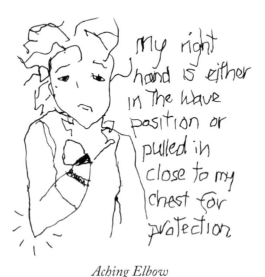

my right hand is either in the wave position or pulled in close to my chest for protection

Aching Elbow

I was to learn as time went on that to have treatment which was beneficial often meant 'discomfort' and at times downright pain, but at least it was better than simply drowning in pain killers and doing nothing. With many injuries it seems that there is a fine line between the pain of keeping moving = **good** and overzealous action which make it more inflamed = **bad**. Again I am not advocating not using pain killers at all, as I would not have been able to endure some weeks without them, but I now know they have to be used in conjunction with early intervention of Occupational Therapy, oedema control, Acupuncture, massage etc. and the earlier, the better! The therapies produce positive results, whereas, pain killers alone just kill pain and from what I have gathered, from others who use them, if you have to take them for long periods, you become used to them and have to up the dosage, or keep changing the variety. I urge you to keep trying to move your affected hand or foot to pro-mote circulation and prevent atrophy of the muscles and bones and hardening of the tissues.

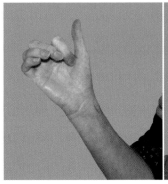 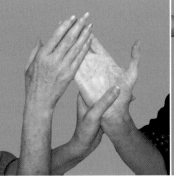 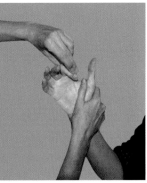

Active Movement   *Passive Movement*   *Passive Movement*

I asked Terry which exercises would be the most beneficial to me and she replied that every movement that I performed would be beneficial, but the action of 'scrubbing' was especially helpful. I have to say at that stage the very notion of trying to grip a brush with my claw like and extremely swollen hand sounded like pure torture. I did try to do it though and when eventually, many months later, I was able to properly grasp the brush I realised how important that kind of stretch is. During those early days I have to admit that a lot of my movements were so minimal that most of the action happened in my head. However even the minimal movement that I was capable of really helped to stretch my wrist and fingers. Again I must stress the importance of doing the exercises that you have been given as many times a day as possible.

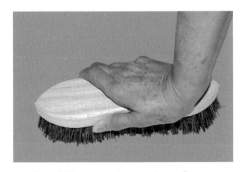 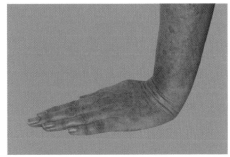

Scrubbing exercises wrist + fingers   *Flat hand stretches wrist + fingers*

No matter how impossible and scary the exercises may seem, provided you stick to the regime your Hand Therapist has given you, they will not harm you. Keep at it, the sooner the better. The longer you leave it the more difficult movement becomes.

Terry explained that there are variations on the scrubbing exercise. It could be done, she said, on a table or some surface which is the right height to enable the position without putting stress on the shoulder.

Later I also found the exercises below really helpful. Even though my hand remained extremely painful and swollen, whenever I walked down the street to the underground or to the high street as a ritual I would try to do the following movements with both hands. As I said they only became fully possible much later in my recovery, but I am putting them here as an illustration of what worked for me. They are really good and I remember the excitement as one by one the three injured fingers managed to make contact with my thumb. I still do this ritual.

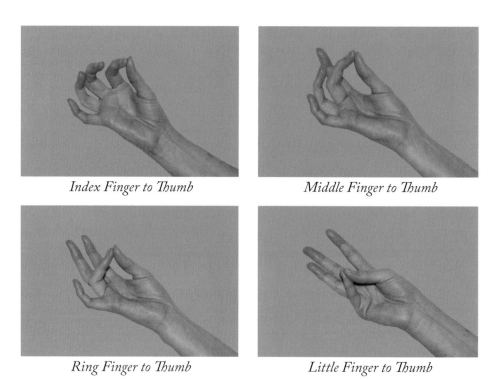

Index Finger to Thumb	*Middle Finger to Thumb*
Ring Finger to Thumb	*Little Finger to Thumb*

Different fractures and other injuries require very different exercises, so do not attempt any of the ones I describe without consulting your Hand Therapist to make sure they correspond to your particular needs! They will give you an exercise routine which will suit you. **This especially applies after surgery!**

Oedema and
Elizabeth's Massage

Meanwhile my friend Elizabeth who was taking an active interest in what was happening to me instinctively felt that gentle hand massage would relieve some of my discomfort. I was not 100% in agreement as the less touching the better as far as I was concerned, but Terry agreed with her and Elizabeth began to give me very, very gentle massages with the tips of her fingers. (I call them massages, but it was more like a very gentle stroking with essential oils.) This was very scary stuff as most of the time even a breeze on my skin was difficult to endure. She asked to come with me to the hand unit so that she could find out what to do and what not to do. Terry explained that the gentle massage was a good idea but it was important to start at the fingertips and work towards the wrist, thereby moving the oedema away from the injury.

What Elizabeth did following that session was extraordinary because sometimes, even when she was stroking my hand really gently I would be crying with the pain because of the skin sensitivity but she persevered, which I felt took some dedication and showed me that she was determined to help me get better. With this gentle massage she kept the circulation going. Her determination to help me never dwindled. It is important to note here that most of the time the pain during those massages was very difficult to cope with, but I know that all this contributed massively to desensitizing the skin, and dispersing some of the oedema, thereby enabling more movement in the long term. I remember one time when she was gently massaging my swollen and rather khaki and bruised hand. A tiny area over one of the knuckles turned pink – it looked normal. We cheered and celebrated and were so excited and even though the pinkness disappeared again we knew there was hope and worked towards getting it back in the whole hand.

I had the benefit of at least twice daily 'massages' and Elizabeth had an instinctive idea of what she was trying to do and knew that it was not just to massage the skin. I was later told by an Occupational Therapist that anecdotal evidence showed that retrograde massage has been noted to be useful, but really needs to be performed at least twice a day for it to have a significant effect.

Here again I urge you to speak to your Hand Therapist before doing anything which may not be the appropriate treatment for your particular case.

The following photographs were done a long time after my recovery and portray the ultimate goals that Elizabeth and I were aiming to achieve. Most of the time within the first 6 months they were only goals and although tiny gains were made sometimes weekly, sometimes longer, many of the movements were completely out of my reach. Elizabeth of course never forced any of the moves, but was persistent and constantly encouraged me to allow her to work on my hands. I will always be grateful for that persistence. I have included the exercises here to re-iterate how important it is to set goals and even when you don't see or feel results immediately, don't give up – keep going!

Elizabeth's massages were approved by the Hand Therapist. Do not do anything like this without consulting your Hand Therapist. They may not be appropriate for your injury.

Women, particularly of a certain age are prone to osteoporosis so please discuss your bone density with your GP and try to get a bone density scan. **Never force any movement.**

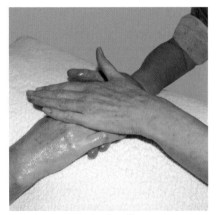

Apply oil

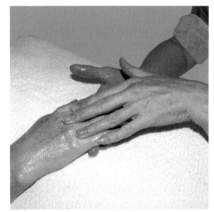

Gently de-sensitise skin

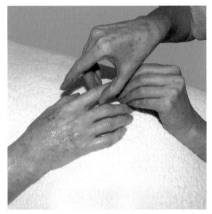

Gently Squeeze Oedema away from Fingertips

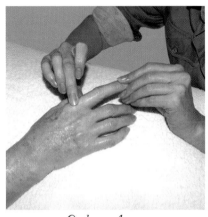

Oedema Away

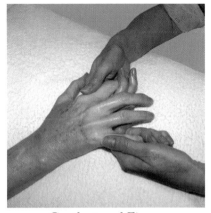

Gently spread Fingers

The above exercises were approved for my particular injury.
It is important that you consult your Hand Therapist before trying any of them!

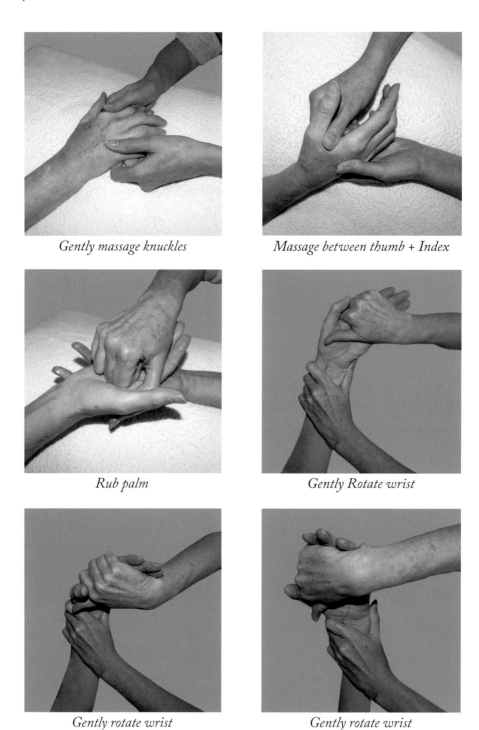

Gently massage knuckles

Massage between thumb + Index

Rub palm

Gently Rotate wrist

Gently rotate wrist

Gently rotate wrist

The above exercises were approved for my particular injury.
It is important that you consult your Hand Therapist before trying any of them!

If you decide to use Essential oils, you will find that they can be very expensive, but if you get carrier oil, like almond oil* you have quite a lot of massage oil fairly cheaply. It is also an idea to go a homeopathic pharmacy and talk to a practitioner. They have given me some very good advice and are patient and helpful and will give you advice over the counter on which oils would be appropriate.

It later became evident that the gentle massage Elizabeth was instinctively doing was similar in its aims to 'retrograde massage'. She was squeezing and pushing the fluid away from the tips of my fingers, up into my hand and away from my injury, whilst gently spreading my fingers and finally rotating my wrist to promote circulation and movement. It worked for me; with Terry's guidance, Elizabeth's innate gift for gentle massage became a crucial element in my recovery.

I kept noticing all the way through that my injury was treated in isolation from the rest of my body and although I had made the decision to always view my body as a whole system it was difficult to do so when each segment of my arm had to be treated in a different medical unit. Although I had pain in my shoulder, the hand unit could only deal with my hand and so on, so with the best will in the world, there was no holistic approach. I think that it is pertinent to mention here that with CRPS, which is thought to be largely a neurological malfunction, it also makes sense to follow through the massage on both hands. The nervous system as with everything else in your body is one system and doesn't end at the edge of the injury. Later, I was lucky enough to have massage to the rest of my body as well. I discovered just how much human touch can help when you are in so much pain. Like the night when I brushed against the wall and Mimi gently held me, Elizabeth's massages were so therapeutic, because of the touch. My body felt so isolated and I was trying so hard to keep myself protected from being bumped, that I shrank away from any physical contact. Those massages were so good in that respect as in many others. Much later I also realised that if CRPS was a nerve condition, trying to restore some sort of balance between the right hand and the left hand was very important and that treating my whole body and not isolating my injured hand was psychologically very healing and made sense.

---

* Not to be used with nut allergies!

By now apart from the extreme swelling and bizarre colour changes, the skin on my hand had become very thin and shiny and there were thick, dark hairs growing across it. I asked Terry about it and she said I ought to make an appointment with the Consultant and talk to her about it. I duly did this and she took my hand in hers and told me that it appeared that I had a condition called RSD or CRPS as is now more widely classified and explained that I had classic symptoms of it. Below is a list of some of the most significant features of this condition as she described them.

- Discoloured and mottled skin with rapid temperature changes.

- Exaggerated pain which is completely out of proportion to the levels expected from the injury.

- An extreme sensitivity to pain where usual and non painful events are felt as pain. For example a breeze over the affected area can be felt as a burn or even sounds can induce pain.

- Cramps, muscle spasms, shooting and stabbing pains which are random and don't correspond to any movement, or contact, or any other stimulus.

- Weakness and an inability to easily move the joints.

- Edema – an accumulation of fluid in the body tissues, general or local. It can be caused by trauma to any part of the body, or by infections, medical conditions, and autoimmune diseases.

- Hair in the affected area grows more rapidly and is thicker and darker.

- The nails harden on the limb in question and initially grow much faster than normal. They can become ridged and malformed.

I felt somewhat vindicated to hear that the array of these familiar symptoms was not just a sign of my impending insanity but well documented symptoms of CRPS.

The Consultant talked a little about it, and explained that although there were several treatments available, none of them singly had actually proved to cure CRPS. What they had discovered, in the case of a limb, was that by keeping it moving as much as possible, you could try to prevent arthritis and osteoporosis and several other conditions that arise out of the bad circulation and general turgidity that are associated with CRPS. Also she told me that approximately 50% of people with this condition get better spontaneously within six months, with or without treatment.

I have to say that considering the odds for recovery were so slim, at no point did she indicate that I should be overly concerned. Instead she seemed sanguine that if I continued my Hand Therapy I could manage the CRPS. She gave me a sense of quiet confidence, as did Terry. For me though, the overriding message I came away with, was that unless I was among the 50% who got better spontaneously, I had as yet an untreatable disorder. It was up to me to work hard.

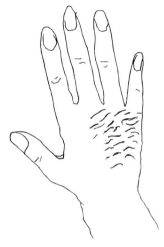

Thick, dark hairs were growing across my hand.

Of course when I got home and looked up CRPS on the net I received a very nasty shock! As people who have the condition know, it is a devastating, degenerative disorder. Early intervention with Occupational or Physiotherapy are very important as in the later stages it is more difficult or sometimes impossible to achieve movement.

Further reading led to my discovering that the first recorded cases of CRPS were made by Silas Weir Mitchell, a doctor treating injured soldiers on the battlefield during the American Civil War where it was called Causalgia.

📖 **For further reading on Silas Weir Mitchell see page 223**

The fact that the first recorded cases were battlefield injuries really made me consider how often it must occur today where guns are prevalent not just in warfare but more and more frequently in civil society.

I also discovered that there are two classifications of CRPS.

CRPS I – Follows an injury to the skin, muscle, ligaments, joints or bone at any site. The injury can be as a result of an accident or surgery. Most commonly it occurs after a bone is broken and immobilised with a splint or a sling, but can occur even after a minor sprain.

CRPS II – Follows partial damage to a nerve in the arm or leg, such as from a gunshot wound or a crush injury. The cluster of painful symptoms that might occur with that sort of high velocity impact are clearly associated with nerve injury.

When I read the accounts written by Silas Weir of soldiers with nerve injuries, and whatever I could find on the net, I felt pretty sure that the 'high velocity' or crush injury criteria was definitely pertinent to me.
When that garden pot weighing between 36 to 40 kilos (80–90 lbs) dropped roughly 75 cm (2 ft 2 inches) onto my flat hand on the floor it must have gathered some velocity.
For myself, I felt as though I had been punched in the gut. As you can see I like to write and draw. I like cooking and gardening and doing a lot of creative things with my hands. This is not to say that it made the diagnosis worse in my case particularly, in fact in retrospect I suppose it gave me a framework of positive goals and targets to work toward, but it was still quite a shock.
At the next appointment with Terry I asked her if she had known about the CRPS. She said she had noticed the signs. I couldn't believe that she had not told me.
"Look." She said. "I don't like to put people in boxes." I protested "But you know I am an 'out of the box' kind of person Terry." "Yes but we are doing all we can be doing anyway and in some cases if people have the diagnosis, they become depressed and since it is so difficult to diagnose, arguably it is better just to keep up the rigorous treatments." I could see her point and had to admit to myself that the new knowledge about the condition was psychologically difficult. It had been scary not knowing why I was in so much pain and now it was scary knowing.

The positive thing about knowing was that I could look at blogs and support group sites. Although I have to admit that was sometimes very frightening in itself. I suppose because the pain was so intense, when I read the most extreme cases and saw photographs of long term CRPS, I imagined myself in those pictures. This was only a temporary response, but on the sleepless nights they turned up in my mind. On the positive side, those same pictures became the driving force of my determination to keep moving and to set about doing my own research programme.

I was astounded at the bravery of some of the bloggers who were so upbeat about living with CRPS/RSD and freely shared their experiences online. This was when I decided to write the book. After my diagnosis I went around bookshops trying to find something about CRPS. There had been one book published in the UK, but unfortunately it was out of print. Having no luck, I resumed my search online. However, I found that sitting at the computer exacerbated the pain in my hand and made it turn more purple, stiff and cramped. Also it is a very slow process using one hand to type, particularly if it is not the dominant one. I imagined there must undoubtedly be a number of people out there experiencing CRPS who would be caught in a vacuum with no information about what they were going through and no way of sharing infor-mation, without computer access. This was now about 6 weeks after my injury and I had only just found out what was causing all these extreme symptoms. I was receiving financial support and moral support from friends and therapists at the hand unit, and I was still extremely traumatised by what was happening to me. I couldn't imagine how others without this support might cope.

I wanted to try and contribute to an awareness about CRPS. I downloaded and printed out Pain Relief Foundation Pamphlet on Complex Regional Pain Syndrome and gave it to friends to read, so they could get an idea of the intensity of the condition.

📖 For the Pain Relief Foundation pamphlet see beginning of book

I think that it shocked everyone at first, but later as I was lucky enough to be able to access therapy, massage and Acupuncture all of which brought a measure of relief, some understandably forgot the seriousness of it. Most would not realise that in general the symptoms persist pretty much day and night. They will forget that unless you are one of the lucky 50%, you are struggling every minute of every day to keep your limb moving to prevent your muscles atrophying and your bones crumbling due to poor circulation. Friends and neighbours *always* asked how I was feeling, but I avoided answering that question truthfully after a while because it was embarrassing for the questioner who was helpless with the information.

With CRPS your limb feels heavy and as though it is full of congealing glue, gumming up all movements. As much as you exercise the one day, you have to continue the next, because most of the time all you are doing is keeping it at bay, but if you stop it gums up again and your limb becomes rigid and very difficult to move. Once during the first few months after my accident I had flu and ran a high temperature and so I just stayed in bed and slept as much as possible. On that occasion my hand became so stiff and painful from lack of movement, that I thought I had lost the battle. But with a lot of hard work courtesy of Elizabeth's absolute determination to keep massaging it and help-ing me to move the joints we always managed to get it moving again.

Please persevere, it is the single most important thing that you can do to help yourself!

The accumulative effect of movement and use really works in the healing process!

So there – no matter how tiring and uncomfortable exercise and movement may be it is absolutely crucial to maintaining circulation. Another gem that Terry passed on to me was that it is not good enough just to exercise the limb, it is crucial to **use it**! Really I can't be more emphatic about this. From the first moment she told me this, I tried to do so, even though the pain was devastat-ing if I even bumped against something. It is very much a slow and steady approach with movement. Even if you are not actually completing the task, follow through the movement with your mind.
One of the 'using' strategies I implemented right from the beginning was when I washed my face in the bath. Even though my wrist and fingers were stiff and swollen and painful, when I was washing around my eyes and cheekbones and nose, I kept my eyes closed and tried to imagine that my right hand which was stiff and claw like and dragged across my skin, was actually moving in the same way as the other one. All the intricate movements which hands perform generally eluded my injured hand, but there were little moments which grew

after time, where I felt a little twinge or imagined for a second that I had feeling in the tips of those fingers. A little later after severe pain in my shoulder kicked in it was impossible to reach up to my face with that arm at all and for some time I was again forced to wash using only my left hand.

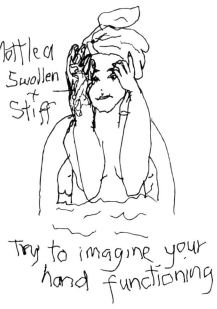

Imagining my hand moving

I was keen to find out what it all looked like under my skin. I wanted to visualise the routes of the pain and what was occurring, so that I could try to move my hand against the destructive effects. I went to my local library and found **The Visual Dictionary of Human Anatomy** (ISBN 0-7513-1063-8).

They are an excellent series and user friendly and simple in their descriptions. Sadly this particular version is now out of print, but for those who are able, you can usually buy used copies online. There are also anatomy books in most libraries. I really recommend them to anyone experiencing painful conditions, because you get to see what your system looks like and have a little more understanding of what your doctor is talking about when they discuss your symptoms etc. Somehow, when I looked at those pictures and focussed on how breathtakingly beautiful the human system is, it spurred me on to look after myself more and eat properly and not pollute my body and actively help it to heal. It is such a perfect design and I think most of the time we can just take that for granted.

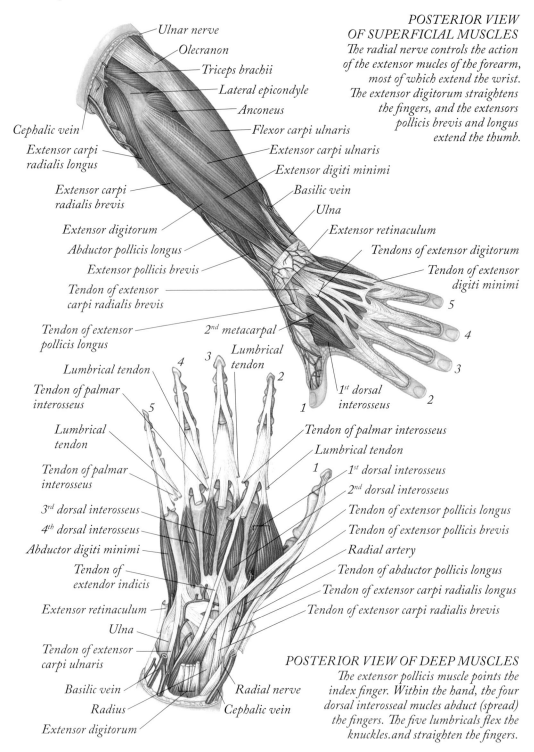

Ulnar nerve
Olecranon
Triceps brachii
Lateral epicondyle
Anconeus
Flexor carpi ulnaris
Cephalic vein
Extensor carpi
radialis longus
Extensor carpi ulnaris
Extensor digiti minimi
Basilic vein
Extensor carpi
radialis brevis
Ulna
Extensor retinaculum
Extensor digitorum
Tendons of extensor digitorum
Abductor pollicis longus
Extensor pollicis brevis
Tendon of extensor
digiti minimi
Tendon of extensor
carpi radialis brevis
5
4
Tendon of extensor
pollicis longus
2nd metacarpal
Lumbrical
tendon
3
Lumbrical tendon
4
2
1st dorsal
interosseus
3
Tendon of palmar
interosseus
5
2
Lumbrical
tendon
1
Tendon of palmar interosseus
Tendon of palmar
interosseus
Lumbrical tendon
1
1st dorsal interosseus
3rd dorsal interosseus
2nd dorsal interosseus
4th dorsal interosseus
Tendon of extensor pollicis longus
Abductor digiti minimi
Tendon of extensor pollicis brevis
Tendon of
extendor indicis
Radial artery
Tendon of abductor pollicis longus
Extensor retinaculum
Tendon of extensor carpi radialis longus
Ulna
Tendon of extensor carpi radialis brevis
Tendon of extensor
carpi ulnaris
Basilic vein
Radial nerve
Radius
Cephalic vein
Extensor digitorum

POSTERIOR VIEW OF SUPERFICIAL MUSCLES
The radial nerve controls the action of the extensor mucles of the forearm, most of which extend the wrist. The extensor digitorum straightens the fingers, and the extensors pollicis brevis and longus extend the thumb.

POSTERIOR VIEW OF DEEP MUSCLES
The extensor pollicis muscle points the index finger. Within the hand, the four dorsal interosseal mucles abduct (spread) the fingers. The five lumbricals flex the knuckles.and straighten the fingers.

By Kind Permission Dorling Kindersley

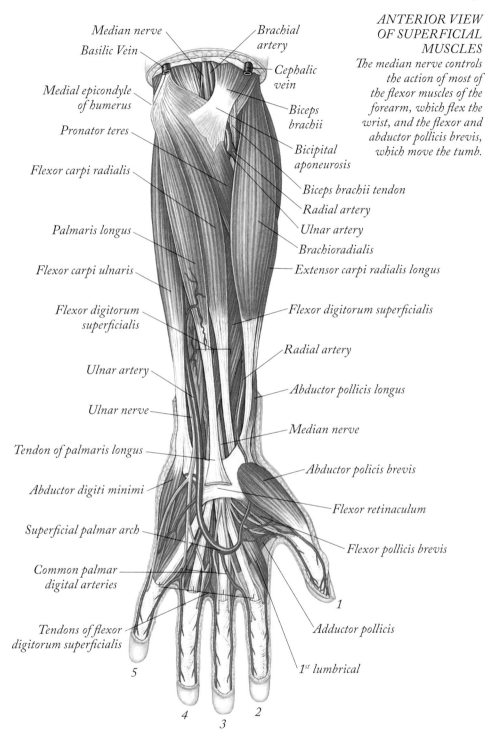

Median nerve

Basilic Vein

Medial epicondyle of humerus

Pronator teres

Flexor carpi radialis

Palmaris longus

Flexor carpi ulnaris

Flexor digitorum superficialis

Ulnar artery

Ulnar nerve

Tendon of palmaris longus

Abductor digiti minimi

Superficial palmar arch

Common palmar digital arteries

Tendons of flexor digitorum superficialis

Brachial artery

Cephalic vein

Biceps brachii

Bicipital aponeurosis

Biceps brachii tendon

Radial artery

Ulnar artery

Brachioradialis

Extensor carpi radialis longus

Flexor digitorum superficialis

Radial artery

Abductor pollicis longus

Median nerve

Abductor policis brevis

Flexor retinaculum

Flexor pollicis brevis

Adductor pollicis

1st lumbrical

5

4

3

2

1

By Kind Permission Dorling Kindersley

Some time after the CRPS diagnosis, I was feeling particularly scared and I called Mimi and she came with me to the Hand Therapy unit and I went home with her afterwards and I stayed the night. I hardly slept a wink and was in non stop agony. I was up very early in the morning and couldn't stop myself sobbing from the pain I was experiencing. I was now really frightened. All my positive thinking and keeping my chin up didn't seem to be helping. I called Elizabeth who said I should come over immediately. Mimi drove me over and dropped me on her way to work.

Elizabeth and Jeff said that I should stay with them for a while. We began a regime of massage three times a day, for at least an hour – sometimes longer. I call it massage, but as I have mentioned before it was really a gentle de-sensitising of the skin and the whole hand.

Elizabeth was so determined to keep my hand moving and that whatever it took to save it she would do, including helping me financially with any treatment. Psychologically again this was a real life raft because now that I knew about the CRPS, I was keen to try and access complimentary treatments including Acupuncture, which Lizzie (Alexander Technique teacher) had suggested. The most important thing now was to ensure that it didn't take over and completely immobilise my hand. Having done some research on the net I was also fully aware that the sorts of treatments that I would want to pursue are largely not available on the NHS. At this point Shal and Rob were still funding my treatment at the private Hand Therapy unit, so Elizabeth's offer gave me the impetus to seek other treatments as well as the Hand Therapy. In my research I was finding many references to multi-disciplinary treatments which in the context of traditional western medicine include quite substantial amounts of pain medications, anti-depressants, nerve blockers etc., in conjunction with Occupational and Physiotherapy. I was interested in seeking a multi-disciplinary regime which excluded the use of too many pain medications and looked more to Diet, Herbal Remedies, Massage, Acupuncture or any other Holistic treatments which would complement the fantastic Hand Therapy.

I continued to go twice a week and before each Hand Therapy session with Terry I would be asked to use the wax bath. (It looks like a deep chip fryer.) The pan contains hot, liquid paraffin wax. The idea is that you submerge your hand in the melted wax and it coats it. After a few seconds you take your hand out, let the wax set for a minute or so, then put it back in and repeat the process a few times until your hand is completely coated with the warm wax. The therapist then places a fine plastic bag over the hand and wraps a towel around the whole thing and allows time for the heat to warm up the hand before beginning therapy. It is a very comforting feeling. It warms and softens the joints so that when the work begins they don't feel so brittle.

You can buy wax baths to use at home. They are fantastically therapeutic and warm the hand very effectively promoting circulation and softening the joints.

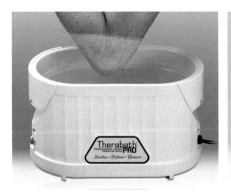 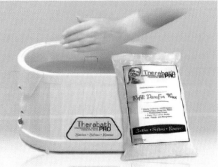

These baths can be used for hands or feet and are also recommended for those who have arthritis or other regional pain syndromes.

📖 **Patterson Medical for wax bath see page 239**

Elizabeth had been doing her own research and had sought advice from an alternative doctor who had helped her manage arthritis for many years. She had recommended that I put my hand into very hot water at least three times a day and keep it there as long as I could to stimulate circulation. She suggested I do this before each of Elizabeth's massages. This was actually very similar to the wax bath before my Hand Therapy with Terry. So before each of our massage sessions I would hold my hand in a jug of very hot water. This was excruciating, but so was everything, so I decided that if it was doing my circulation a favour, I would bite the bullet and do it. I have continued to do that to promote circulation and it really works for me. I use a tall plastic picnic jug that I had bought at the supermarket. I stand it on a low stool so that I am able to easily get my hand into it without straining my shoulder. When it comes out I dry it carefully and wrap it in a dry towel for a few minutes before we begin the massage.

Please do not do this without discussing it with your Hand Therapist or doctor this may not be good for your condition!

During the first few sessions with Elizabeth I found myself focussing too much on my hand, so I didn't relax. I always believe that laughter is the best medicine and so we decided that while she massaged I would read to us. I love Carl Hiaasen. I have put his web address below. I had been given his newest book (at that time) **Skinny Dip** and so that was what we read. Jeff would come into the room to see what was going on and we would be screaming with laughter. I believe that this laughter contributed positively to my emotional state at that time. Carl Hiaasen is a master of farce. You either love him or hate him. His sense of humour is very dark. His books are widely available in bookshops or for those online at **www.carlhiaasen.com**

It was during this time whilst reading out loud that I began to discover how difficult it is to manage a paperback book with one hand. I got cramp in my uninjured thumb and turning pages was a nightmare. I later went out looking for book holders which would be helpful, but although there are some which work, the better ones are heavy and cumbersome or the light ones have complicated mechanisms to deal with using only one hand. It was this experience and the fact that I am an avid reader that informed the decision to produce this book in hardback in the larger format. It means that it can be rested on the reader's lap or on a table and the print size is appropriate. The pages stay open! I would like the reader to be able to read and peruse the anatomical illustrations without having to juggle the book.

In spite of all the care I was receiving, my hand was still very swollen, the skin was tight, shiny, and a sort of khaki colour, with grey blotches of varying shades. It would quickly change to a mottled purple and pale cold blue. It changed colour like some exotic creature on a David Attenborough programme. There was no definition of bones or knuckles, even my little wrist bone had disappeared into a thick swelling. The pinkness on my knuckle that Elizabeth and I had noticed came and went. The sensations ranged from freezing, like a sort of frostbite, to something resembling being singed with a blow torch. I had shooting pains up and down my arm and sometimes from my shoulder deep into my elbow and there were cramps and contractions. Actually at that time I was wide eyed with pain most hours in the day and night.

I had not done much about sorting out some Acupuncture, but another friend Gioia, who is an oracle as far as 'where to go for what', pointed me in the direction of a certain Dr. Gang Zhu, (a member British Register of

Complementary Practitioners – BRCP) who practices in a health clinic in Notting Hill Gate. I called him and arranged an appointment. I was so impressed at my first meeting with him; when I showed him the x rays, he told me that he had been in orthopaedics in China and he was able to make some pertinent comments about the fracture. After an assessment, he said that he felt he could help me, but wished that I had come earlier, as the hand was now very fibrous and so it would take some time. What he proposed was five weeks of intensive Acupuncture, twice a week, then once a week, for five weeks and then we would re-assess. Unfortunately this was not going to be funded by the NHS. Again because of financial support I felt very lucky to have the opportunity to try this course of action. It is my hope that the NHS will fund more Acupuncture in the future as it is such an effective treatment and as it turned out it was perfect for me at that time.

I want to be very clear about Acupuncture for those who have a fear of needles. The so called 'needles' are as fine as hairs and are <u>not</u> stiff like sewing needles. Mostly you don't feel them at all, going in or coming out. Before I had Acupuncture, I imagined them to be like hat pins. They really are more like hairs than needles. Always make sure that your practitioner is regulated.

📖 **For details on The Institute for Complementary and Natural Medicine (ICNM) see page 203**

Dr. Zhu began treating me that night and I have to say, because of the stiffness of my hand, which was still excessively swollen, gummed up around the knuckles, and extremely sensitive to touch, it was difficult at first for him to get the needles in. Whereas often Acupuncture is not too painful that first session was quite uncomfortable, because one or two points between my fingers were very tight, due to the CRPS, the scarring and the nature of the crush injury. However, it released an enormous emotional energy and I lay there with tears running down my cheeks, filling up my ears. I felt really stupid. I decided to walk back to Elizabeth's and Jeff's and as soon as I was out of the centre, I burst into tears and sobbed out loud all the way back, which was about a ten minute walk. I know that this is not uncommon with Acupuncture as it unblocks 'channels'. I also think weeping can be a healthy thing to do, as I have already said. Over the next five weeks I attended Acupuncture with Dr. Zhu and found it so relaxing lying quietly in soft lighting while the Acupuncture needles did their job. I was also given some treatment points for sleep, which gave me a couple of restful night's sleep every week. I was very grateful for that. Elizabeth, as she continued to massage my hand several times a day commented after the second week that the gummed up area around my knuckles felt as though it was breaking down. This became even more evident over the next eight weeks and both Elizabeth and the Occupational Therapists, commented on the marked difference of the restrictions in movement. I have to make very clear here that CRPS is so powerful, that significant changes observed by those treating it might not be obvious to the sufferer. The array of painful sensations which continuously bombard the injured limb tend to mask any progress. Sometimes even when I felt there was significant progress within a short time those gains would disappear. This is why I believe that it is so important not to expect the work you do to have instant results, but to keep going. It is a long journey and the accumulative work that you do does eventually pay off. After the first five weeks attending twice a week, I attended the next five once weekly.

As a result of the enthusiasm shown by both Elizabeth and the OT's (Occupational Therapists) I was keen to keep going at the end of the ten weeks. I was a bit disappointed when Dr. Zhu explained that at this point we should halt the Acupuncture and I should make a follow up appointment in four weeks to reassess. He also suggested that I should try to see a physiotherapist for my shoulder.

I believe that the work that Dr. Zhu did on my hand at that point in conjunction with the massage and OT was pivotal to me still being able to move it today. Dr. Gang Zhu is a registered member of ICNM.

What works for one person does not always work for another and the decision to use Acupuncture or any therapy should be made with as much caution as a decision to take medication. I urge anyone who may be thinking of using this treatment to consult their Hand Therapist or GP and contact (ICNM) or other recognised institutions who have lists of regulated Acupuncturists. There will always be some unscrupulous 'practitioners' whose activities are not regulated and who could cause damage to your health. Make every effort to avoid them and find a practitioner who has a track record.

📖 **For contacts of registered Acupuncturists see pages 203 and 211**

Some believe that Acupuncture by its nature is invasive and therefore can aggravate the CRPS so consult a health professional. For me this was not the case.

I was beginning to develop a multidisciplinary treatment regime – where several disciplines are used concurrently. As the patient, using this approach, you have to be determined to stay with a number of programmes and work hard at them. Sometimes when you feel as though you have made progress one minute it can seem to be all swept away the next.

Just to illustrate how strong the CRPS is, even with the massage, Hand Therapy, Acupuncture and the use of Ibuprofen and Paracetamol, I was still having shocking cramps and shooting nerve pains and I could never make it through the night without waking in searing pain. The exception was the couple of nights a week after I had Acupuncture. Proponents of drugs may use this as an example as to why conventional medication works better, but I am prepared to forgo the quick fix or instant temporary relief for the possibility of a well rounded long term solution. Added to the fact that strong painkillers are known to cause constipation and I had no intention of adding that to my list of symptoms. What I really didn't need at this stage was a 'plumbing' problem.

At the back of my mind was always the original diagnosis when I was told that 50% of people don't recover from CRPS. I was determined that I would find a way to keep my hand moving in the hope that eventually it would recover sufficiently for me to live a 'normal' life again. In spite of that determination there were moments when I contemplated that maybe I wouldn't get better and that my hand was in the throes of dying. That may sound dramatic, but pain at the sort of level that CRPS delivers is pretty all consuming and gives rise to a number of frightening concepts. I had also read many accounts on the web of some sufferers being so unable to cope with the pain that they opted for amputation or of others even committing suicide. These related to American experiences.

Thankfully I was surrounded by supportive friends and was receiving excellent treatments, so I was always able to hold onto a positive attitude. After about three weeks of Acupuncture the extreme swelling began to abate a bit and by the end of the five weeks it was significantly less swollen than it had been when we started.

The Hand Therapists (by now I was seeing other therapists as well as Terry) all agreed that there was a marked improvement although I still had to wear the oedema glove to manage the swelling.

CRPS II, which is the one I believe I had, is said to be the result of damage to a peripheral nerve.

Peripheral Nerve – any nerve which is outside of the central nervous system. The central nervous system is comprised of the brain and spinal cord, which are located in and protected by the skull and the vertebral column. Peripheral Nerves are the ones in the rest of the body.

CRPS II, in a general definition as I see it is as follows:
- The nerves send messages to the brain, which is then able to take appropriate actions. When an injury occurs, alarm signals are sent and the brain alerts the rest of the system, swelling occurs and pain ensues. The injured person or others will then try as much as they can to protect the affected area by covering it, supporting it, applying pressure to stop bleeding, or whatever first aid is appropriate.

- In normal situations, these alarm signals will die down as the injury is treated and various aches and pains and bruising will be present during the healing process. With CRPS, the messages going to the brain are scrambled and it is almost like 'Groundhog Day' where the main alarm message about the injury plays over and over again, triggering pain and causing oedema to accumulate at the location.

A nutritionist described to me the lymph system and its function. From what I understood, it is an incredibly intricate system of vessels running throughout your body, drawing off and processing excess fluids which are lost from the blood vessels and capillaries and collect in the tissues. He asked me to imagine a very fine lace glove. This is what the lymph system would resemble in my hand. "It lies" he said "just under the skin".

The following illustration corresponds absolutely to his description.

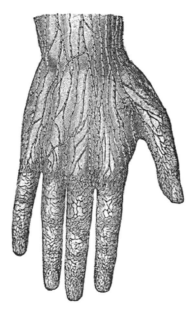

Lymphatic vessels of the dorsal surface of the hand.
Henry Gray (1825–1861). Anatomy of the Human Body. 1918.

I imagine when I had the accident, mine became damaged and, because of the 'stuck record' syndrome of the CRPS, the oedema was pumping into the region, but had nowhere to go and so was collecting and congealing, creating a gumming up of my joints and all the soft tissue.

Usually after an initial trauma, as healing begins, and this usually begins very quickly, the whole system will work together to mend the affected area. In the case of CRPS where these major message functions and drainage systems are malfunctioning, it can trigger other unpleasant health problems. These can include changes to bones and muscle atrophy, not to mention a range of painful symptoms, including cramps, muscle spasms, stabbing pains, temperature changes and extreme skin sensitivity to the extent that even a breeze on the area will feel like fire or frostbite. All of the above symptoms I have mentioned earlier.

As soon as you are able to move the affected area (In the case of a limb, or hand, or foot) do so and continue to do so. Sometimes it is exhausting to keep going, because you may be able to achieve significant movement and then within an hour, or less, it will revert right back to its rigid state.

Please do not give up! Please keep going!

In all the journal entries and records that I came across, dating back to the American Civil war where Causalgia (CRPS) is discussed, oedema management is deemed to be one of the most important factors in treating the disorder. I know that for me while the oedema remained, so did the pain and the restrictions in movement.

Mirror Therapy

During the course of Occupational Therapy I was introduced to Amy, a Hand Therapist at the clinic who was trained to do visual feedback therapy. For me this was quite miraculous, and with the following explanation in mind I hope to be able to encourage anyone having problems moving a limb, to try it. It is simple and doesn't cost the world and is something you can do on your own. The technique of mirror work was developed by Vilayanur S. Ramachandran to help alleviate 'phantom limb' pain. Amputees can still experience often vivid and painful sensations in the location of a limb that has been amputated.

📖 **For further reading on Phantom Limb Pain see page 185**

The concept behind mirror work as I have understood it is that since the messages to the brain have been scrambled by a trauma to the nerves, what is happening is much like an electrical short circuit. Mechanisms are firing but the signals are confused. If the brain can be tricked visually into thinking the injury has healed, there is a possibility that some of the scrambled messages can be untangled bringing some movement and some relief. The eye is one of the sensory receptors passing messages directly to the brain. In this case the visual aspect of the injury.

What follows is a description of my experience of visual feedback at that time when my hand was so immobile and in so much pain.

If I put both hands out in front of me and try to do certain simple movements, I am aware of the inability of my right hand to complete some of them.
I can see and feel the symptoms of the CRPS. I am also conscious because of the weeks of pain, the x ray images and the medical diagnosis that there are serious problems occurring in my hand which preclude 'normal' function and movement. There is a "can't" aspect to the exercise.

If I close my eyes and do the movements, I am still aware of the shortcomings of my right hand.

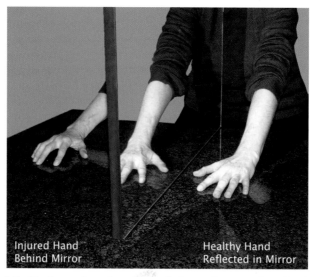

Injured Hand
Behind Mirror

Healthy Hand
Reflected in Mirror

Visual feedback requires that the limb that is being reflected is healthy.

If, however, I have my injured hand behind a mirror and my uninjured one lined up in a position that the image in the mirror conveys two healthy hands and I try to do identical movements with both hands and focus on the reflection I become convinced that I am seeing both hands functioning well. Remember your eyes are sensory receptors sending their version of the situation to your brain. I know that at first it sounds dubious, but I can only advise those with an injured hand to try it, it really works. I worked briefly with the Hand Therapist who was using mirror therapy (probably about three or four sessions). They didn't last for more than about 10 minutes at a time. Amy encouraged me to try using objects with different textures, to stimulate sensory reflexes. She would give me a pom pom for each hand, or thera putty or sponges. It felt like magic to me. I could definitely feel a shift of some sort in my injured hand within seconds.

Some exercises I was shown for my therapy regime:

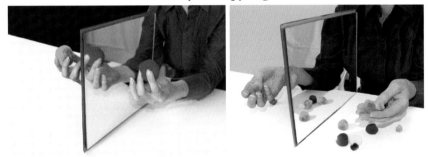

The use of craft shop pom poms help to stimulate sensation

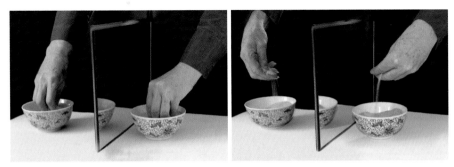

Using fine sand in a bowl creates sensation by literally feeling the texture of it. By trying to lift the sand out of the bowl sensation is again stimulated as it drains through the fingers.

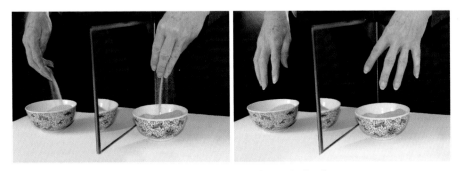

*As the last sand drains out through the fingers,
the action of flicking the fingers open stimulates circulation.*

The exercises above with the sand* can be done using rice. It is about stimulating sensation.

---

* I used sand from the pet shop, sold for use in birdcages. It is river sand, so be cautious if you are prone to allergies. It was certainly fine for me.

I found using the sand had profound sensory results, even long after my CRPS had gone. The tiny grains of sand stimulate the senses in the hand and fingers. Also the sand or rice exercises are best done standing and are useful with or without the mirror.

Try not to use movements that will strain your injured hand when doing mirror work. Use active exercises. If you do strain your hand the resulting discomfort over rides visual feedback, the illusion is destroyed and defeats the purpose. Over a period of time using different therapies, I was able to instigate more and more movement. In the early stages, I just did small movements regularly. Much, much later in my recovery, the exercise I liked the best was to put on some cool jazz or classical music and move my hands in fluid movements which exercise and stretch the wrist and knuckles and fingers. The resonance of the music calms the nerves.

I was so impressed by the positive results with the mirror box at the Hand Unit that I asked my friend Vic if he could make one for me. He made it and I began using it straight away and I know that out of all the therapies and devices, I really felt immediate results from my mirror work.

📖 **For a controlled study of Visual feedback see page 173**

FROZEN SHOULDER

I was now almost four months into the trauma and found that my shoulder was becoming more and more stiff and painful. Dr. Zhu, the Acupuncturist had been treating me for this. Our first five weeks of intensive treatment had come to an end and I was now seeing him once a week. He continued to give me treatment to help me sleep and on the nights after Acupuncture I slept better, but on other nights the pain in my hand and now my shoulder woke me up at least once a night. Dr. Zhu again suggested that I should try to access some Physiotherapy for my shoulder in addition to his treatment. Unfortunately this proved to be an impossible feat.

This additional location of extreme discomfort caused real problems because I needed to keep my arm and hand moving as much as possible to try and counteract the CRPS, but the shoulder was so painful that it became very difficult. I did find ways to relieve some of the pain for short periods, but they were at best uncomfortable. I noticed that some of the muscles close to my armpit felt as though they were contracting and I wanted to stretch them.

If you look at the picture on the following page, I can explain how I tried to do this by using the actual names of the muscles. The image covers much more than the shoulder, but is at the perfect angle to demonstrate what I am trying to describe. Before the accident I had very little idea of the way anything looked under my skin, but now I relied heavily on anatomical drawings to inform me and in this case to find ways to try and relieve the pain in my shoulder.

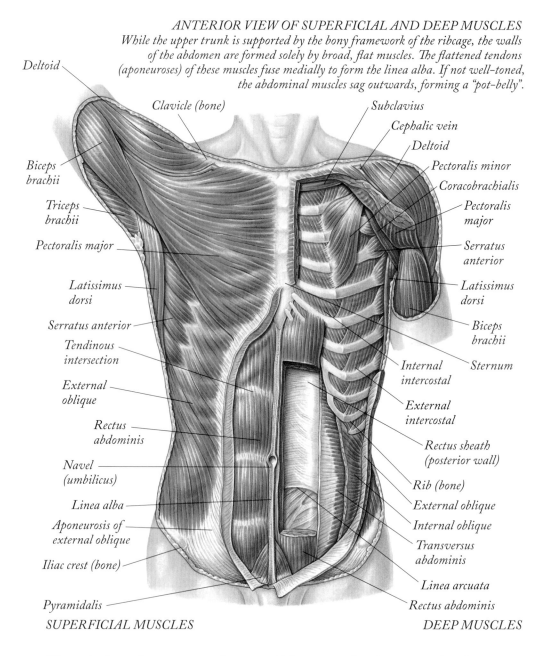

ANTERIOR VIEW OF SUPERFICIAL AND DEEP MUSCLES
*While the upper trunk is supported by the bony framework of the ribcage, the walls
of the abdomen are formed solely by broad, flat muscles. The flattened tendons
(aponeuroses) of these muscles fuse medially to form the linea alba. If not well-toned,
the abdominal muscles sag outwards, forming a "pot-belly".*

Deltoid

Clavicle (bone)

Subclavius

Cephalic vein

Deltoid

Pectoralis minor

Coracobrachialis

Biceps
brachii

Pectoralis
major

Triceps
brachii

Serratus
anterior

Pectoralis major

Latissimus
dorsi

Latissimus
dorsi

Serratus anterior

Biceps
brachii

Tendinous
intersection

Internal
intercostal

Sternum

External
oblique

External
intercostal

Rectus
abdominis

Rectus sheath
(posterior wall)

Navel
(umbilicus)

Rib (bone)

Linea alba

External oblique

Aponeurosis of
external oblique

Internal oblique

Transversus
abdominis

Iliac crest (bone)

Linea arcuata

Pyramidalis

Rectus abdominis

SUPERFICIAL MUSCLES

DEEP MUSCLES

Ok so look at the arm stretching up. My ***triceps brachii*** seemed to have con-
tracted and I couldn't reach upwards, or sideways, or backwards, or even across
the front of me to zip my trousers. Attempting any of the above just resulted
in the most cutting pain deep in my shoulder. I found that soaking in a hot
bath with a teacup of Epson salts (roughly 200–300 grams) helped me to feel
less tense and more able to try and gently move my shoulder. Then when my

body was warm, using some oil (either essential oil or even baby oil) I would pour some into my hand and try to massage the muscle. I would do this for a while gently stretching with long firm strokes the *triceps brachii* and the *latissimus dorsi* in the hope that by stimulating the muscles and stretching them even slightly I might be able to prevent it all becoming more and more rigid and immobilised. The other source of a dark pain was at the point where the *biceps brachii* meets the *deltoid*. It felt like it had knotted and was cramping. This point was a little more sensitive to massage, but again after doing so for as long as possible, making sure to keep the arm warm, it did feel better than just keeping it immobilised. I also think that by finding the actual locations of the various pains and trying to soothe them, it helped me to keep in mind the whole system and not view each symptom in isolation. This was quite good for me psychologically. I have to stress this activity was not a miraculous instant cure, in fact, like most of the exercises that I was doing, it just gave minor relief, but it did give that, so I kept it up.

My mother had always used Epsom salt baths as a treatment after an accident involving sprains or broken bones, or in the case of older members of the family: a good soak after a long day. I used them on the basis of being brought up with them, but when I looked them up I found on the 'Neurological Associates Pain Management' website the following piece of information which seemed to confirm my mother's old fashioned remedy and some! There was also always a bottle of Milk of Magnesia in our house.

Hyperosmolar therapy refers to the fact that some chemicals such as magnesium sulphate (Epsom salt) help to reduce the neuroinflammation, swelling, as well as flexor spasm of the small joints. This is achieved by the patient taking an Epsom salt bath in the bathtub or taking Milk of Magnesia, no more that one to two ounces a day. The magnesium being a calcium channel blocker as well as a very strong osmotic chemical, which extracts the calcium and facilitates the inflow of calcium through the skin. This form of treatment is very effective to counteract the neuroinflammatory edema of CRPS/RSD, as well as relieving the patient's pain.

By Kind Permission of Neurological Associates Pain Management Centre Vero Beach, Florida, USA

www.rsdrx.com

I later found that Epsom salt can be used to exfoliate. If you put a couple of tablespoons into a bowl and add a few drops of water (not enough to dissolve the salts completely) take it up in your hands and rub over the intended area and then wash off. After being in a plaster cast the skin becomes dry and flaky, so this treatment is very helpful to rub away the dead skin. I find it works wonders as an exfoliant on my face, though this is good for my skin it may be too abrasive for others.

You will see all the way through this book that I keep saying "later I discovered," or "much later a doctor told me" because in those early days it was quite difficult to find anything out. I felt quite scared because I had read that little is known about CRPS and it was certainly my experience, with the exception of the Hand Therapy unit, but of course they don't treat the shoulder which in my case was now becoming a new focus of torment.

Much later, long after I had been diagnosed rather distractedly as having Frozen Shoulder I was told by a more interested doctor that the condition is very common after a hand injury and in the past was routinely referred to as 'shoulder hand syndrome'. Even later I discovered that it has been noted to sometimes accompany CRPS in the hand. Obviously I knew that there was a strong possibility that my shoulder might suffer as a result of the immobility of my hand, but I felt cheated that I did not have that information from the beginning. I had felt quite frightened at this new pain because at first I thought the CRPS had moved to my shoulder and psychologically this was not good. Actually, finally (about five months later, after an MRI scan) I was diagnosed not with frozen shoulder but Subachromial Bursitis. Structurally a completely different condition but displaying similar symptoms.

However around this time I was told it was **adhesive capulitis** (medical name for frozen shoulder) so I did some research and was depressed to discover that this new condition could last up to two years and had three distinctive stages. The most important thing to know about it is, as I have described previously, extremely sharp pains occur deep in the shoulder when attempting to move the arm in some directions.

For me this proved a problem because I needed to keep my arm and hand moving to try and promote circulation and prevent my hand from becoming stiff and even more incapacitated than it already was. I assumed I was in stage one, which is apparently a time when the shoulder can be worked on with physiotherapy or exercise regimes. These are not proved to completely cure or stop the condition in its tracks, but help to maintain a range of movements which is always a good thing.

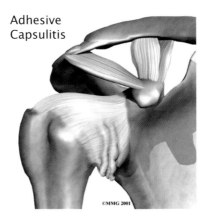

Frozen Shoulder

If you suffer from a painful shoulder, try as early as possible to get a diagnosis and a referral for physiotherapy.

I sadly was unable to do this but luckily I had discovered the self help massages described earlier, and there were Dr. Zhu's fantastic Acupuncture sessions. Not long after this in that well functioning Occupational Therapy Unit described earlier I found they displayed all sorts of information leaflets for the benefit of their clients. Their stock of information is regularly replenished and always really helpful. I found information produced by ARC/ARUK formerly Arthritis Research Campaign now called Arthritis Research UK.

They have a range of very useful information booklets which they invite readers to contribute to and update. They are generous in their information <u>and</u> have one on RSD/CRPS and one on Painful Shoulder (Frozen Shoulder). If you are using a computer I recommend you visit their website.

They talk about all aspects of living with arthritis which, as those who have CRPS might already know, is something which can develop quite rapidly with the condition. Even if you don't have arthritis these booklets are full of helpful tips. They include information on osteoporosis, fibromyalgia, complementary therapies and many other painful conditions.

📖 **For details on Arthritis Research UK see page 197**

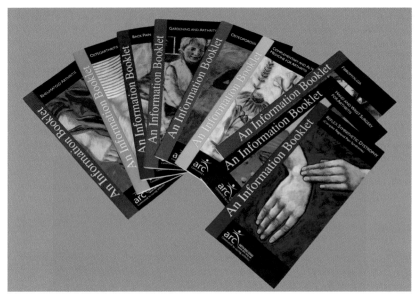

Arthritis Research UK Booklets cover many different conditions

Meanwhile I had discovered with the advent of the 'frozen shoulder' my wave position sleeping arrangements had to change. I could no longer assume the wave position in bed, it was too painful. Later I would discover the V shaped pillow (mentioned on page 36 and 37). This pillow can be strategically placed to give perfect support for an injured shoulder and at the same elevate the arm and hand. For me though at that stage I was still stacking many pillows to achieve this.

The V pillow is one of the most important discoveries I made in terms of pain control when trying to sleep. Unfortunately for me I didn't discover it until eight months later. Below are some drawings of positions and exercises that I worked out to keep my elbow, wrist and hand moving in the hope of preventing any joint problems. I have included the V pillow in the drawings. The V pillow gives support to the shoulder so that the tension is taken off it

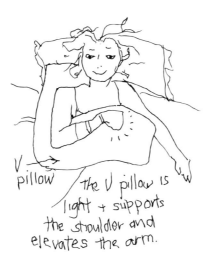

V pillow / The V pillow is light + supports the shoulder and elevates the arm.

and prevents it from flopping backwards, which is excruciating. It did occur to me that the shoulder problems may have stemmed from the unusual posture of the wave position, but since a sling was impossible for me because of the pain, I had very little choice. I found that doing a lot of hand and arm exercises were much more comfortable when lying in bed. So on the many occasions when I woke in the night I would use the opportunity to promote movement.

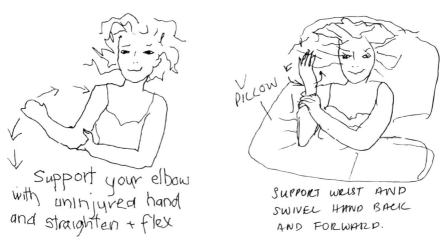

Support your elbow with uninjured hand and straighten + flex

V PILLOW

SUPPORT WRIST AND SWIVEL HAND BACK AND FORWARD.

Exercises for arm and hand in bed

I have spoken to others with CRPS who have also found exercising in bed at night or whilst lying down is much more comfortable for the hand, wrist or arm. This is probably because by doing it like this your limb is never hanging down and the elbow is well supported.

Around this time it was obvious to me that my situation was going to be long term. I had managed the immediate emergency with the amazing help of Shal and Elizabeth, but it would been entirely unrealistic to expect these wonderful friends to continue paying for me to be treated privately. As scared as I still was, I felt confident that now, with all the work that I had been doing and with my medical file recording all the treatments, I would be perceived as less of a nuisance and more as a pro-active patient, willing to work hard at my recovery. Sadly this was not the case. Mmmmm.

I informed the private clinic where I was having the Hand Therapy that I would no longer be able to keep up the private treatment. They prepared me a home programme to continue with what we had been doing. Terry wrote me a detailed clinical update to present to the Senior OT at the NHS Occupational Therapy Unit. The clinical history included the whole history, beginning with that first day, four months previously when she had made the first thermoplastic splint for me. She included all the OT routines and my record of progress. During discussions with the OT's I had found out that the consultant who had been treating me headed a fracture clinic at a hospital closer to where I live, so I decided to try and attend that one as I liked the idea of the continuity. I knew that as a patient I could elect the hospital of my choice using the Choose and Book system. I was told I would require a referral from my GP for this.

'Seamless Transitions!'

On 21st October I went to see a doctor at my local GP surgery. I told him about what had been happening and that I required a referral for the fracture clinic. It is at a hospital closer to where I live than the original one where I had gone as an emergency patient and then as an outpatient. I am entitled to make that choice. For choices go to **www.nhs.uk** or ask your Chemist, GP or Library for the contact number of your local NHS Services.

After perusing all my records on his computer, the GP informed me that the only record that he had regarding my accident, was one note from the original fracture clinic saying that I had attended accident and emergency for a fractured hand. So I would need to get a letter from the fracture clinic and one from the private Consultant outlining the treatment I had been receiving and a diagnosis of the CRPS. I understood that requirement completely.

📖 **For Tips and Health Information see page 167**

I had brought a download of the Pain Relief Foundation's Pamphlet on CRPS. I asked the GP if he knew what CRPS was and he said "NO." He skimmed the page and took up my hand and began to touch the skin, "Does this hurt?" he pressed "No, not in the way described in the article, because I have been having Acupuncture…" He pressed another spot "Here, does that hurt?" actually that time it was pretty excruciating, but I could see where this was going and I realised that my 10 minute slot was going to end shortly and I hadn't achieved anything, so I abandoned the idea of trying to tell him of the achievements resulting from the Acupuncture, Occupational Therapy and Elizabeth's gentle massage. I had also hoped to be able to discuss with him that I had considered applying for incapacity benefit. It would certainly have helped to alleviate my financial situation and my dependency on my friends. I was resisting applying because I was worried that psychologically it would not be a good thing. I had no doubt in my own mind that my hand left me incapable of working, but for me part of the healing process was to be as positive as I could. To apply for the benefit I would have had to emphasise all that was negative about my injury, and that was the opposite of what I was trying to do. That is not to say that I wasn't racked with perpetual and withering pain, but I had tried to keep active and doing things to stop myself from feeling depressed about what was happening to me. Sadly I had to also abandon this important conversation as I felt it would unnecessarily clutter our pressured appointment.

So instead I told him that the Hand Therapist I had been seeing (Terry) had mentioned that I should have a bone density test, because one of the symptoms of CRPS is a rapid thinning of the bones, so I asked him for a referral for one. He seemed to get agitated when I mentioned this, but said that he would do the referral, but that it could take months. I knew that this could be a possibility in the NHS. Before I left he handed me a prescription for anti depressants. I left feeling anxious and frustrated, but confident that at least I had secured a referral for a bone density test. I immediately wrote to the consultant I had seen at the private clinic asking her to send a letter to my GP outlining my medical situation. (When I say wrote, it sounds easy – I sat at the computer using one finger, with my freezing cold hand constantly changing colour and cramping and contracting.)

From then on I resolved to write letters to confirm any requests for referrals and keep all the copies for my file. I knew that this would probably make me very unpopular, but I already felt as though I was viewed as a nuisance so I had little to lose and much to gain health wise by prompting a recorded response to my requests. I also made an appointment with the original Fracture Clinic so that I could try to make sure that all my records were intact and available to all those who needed to see them. This would be particularly important when I got the referral I had requested to the clinic closer to me suggested by the Consultant. I felt that I needed to clear up any confusion that may have arisen because of my move to private health care and then back into the NHS.

Keep copies of **everything**. Doctors and administrators come and go, but it is important for you to keep a record of your progress. It saves time at appointments and if things get lost, you know exactly when they were last seen.

📖 **For some NHS patient information see page 167**

I have also realised after speaking to healthcare professionals that it is very frustrating to be faced with a patient experiencing intractable pain and particularly something like CRPS which is such an unknown entity. They can feel helpless especially if the patient has tried pain medication and continues to experience the overwhelming pain. I can also see that if the patient (like me) avoids even the pain medication, it can be even more frustrating. I hope that this book may reach some of those health workers and maybe present some other options to suggest to their patients particularly the importance of movement, early occupational and any other forms of therapy which will support their recovery in a positive way.

I attended my appointment at the original NHS Fracture Clinic and was the last patient to be seen, by someone who looked as though he just wanted to get it over with. I had been sitting for two and a half hours in a large waiting room full of patients, with a television blaring out mindless cartoons which nobody was watching. My nerves were feeling very frayed by the treble tone of the TV as one by one the other patients were called and the room emptied. It occurred to me that I had been left till last as punishment for going private. I felt quite emotional at that point but decided that at least I had the option of healthcare, unlike millions of others on the planet and so I just bit the bullet and waited. I watched as all the nurses left for the night and the reception closed and all the Doctors left and was just about to give up when a Doctor came out with my file and called me in.

I explained that I wanted to try to update my records and that I had been diagnosed as having CRPS. When I saw that what I had just said made no impact at all, I wished that I had brought Terry's record of my treatment to show him, but it was addressed to the Senior Occupational Therapist at the OT unit.

The doctor seemed irritable and said that he could refer me to a pain clinic, but that I need not hold my breath about getting an appointment any day soon. He also said he could not update my records without a report from who ever had been treating me privately.

I was overwhelmed with disappointment and felt tears welling in my eyes and just wanted to get out of there since he had hardly even looked at me since I came in. I reached for my coat and was paralyzed with pain in my shoulder, which he did notice and asked me "Can you move this way, that way, this way?" he moved his hand and arm around to demonstrate. When I tried to do the movements they were all completely impossible for me and were very painful. He then announced "You have frozen shoulder." I asked him to note on my records that he had diagnosed this and for a referral to a Pain Clinic.

If someone diagnoses a condition in that way, ask them if there are any other conditions which could display the same symptoms. If so, would treatment for the one be detrimental for the other. I am not talking about medication, because the standard treatment offered it seems for absolutely everything is a cortisone injection. I suspect this may be more so in people over 50. I have heard positive and negative reports about cortisone from various friends who have had it. Sometimes it is an instant cure and the condition goes away and never comes back, but often it returns within 6 months and another injection is required. Ask about physiotherapy, about whether there are scans available to prove the diagnosis. Ask them to explain what the term means and how it creates the pain. Try to inform yourself about what is happening to you.

📖 **For NHS advice on how to make the most out of a medical appointment** **see page 170**

HERBS, MASSAGE, MEDITATION AND ROCKS

Elizabeth and Jeff moved out of London at this point and although I was still sometimes on my knees in agony I was determined to take control of my medical destiny. I missed Elizabeth and our times together and all the massages. Elizabeth suggested I find someone else in London to keep up the gentle massage on my hand and she would fund it.

I began attending the NHS Occupational Therapy Department which I have described before and discontinued seeing Terry. It was a very smooth transition because of Joseph's (OT) excellent treatments and Terry's careful and comprehensive record of the treatment I had received. I looked forward to going for therapy because all my questions were answered fully and often I went home with a pamphlet or a web address to get more details regarding something that I had enquired about. I found all of this very re-assuring.

Conveniently for me Marilena, who is a herbalist and who practises massage with healing oils, lives in my neighbourhood. It could not have been better. Now Elizabeth had moved out of town Marilena agreed to take on the rather delicate task of working on my hand. I was scared, because Elizabeth knew all about my hand and the pain and how much pressure to apply and in some ways had instinctively devised a series of very gentle movements which relieved the pressure between my knuckles. I needn't have been concerned, because Marilena immediately did a lot of research on the CRPS, consulted others who had experience of the condition, and mixed up creams and oils with St John's Wort, (hypericum) calendula and other herbs and we began our twice weekly meetings.

> If you are referred for Hand Therapy or physiotherapy after surgery or an accident, attend as many sessions as you can and take advantage of everything the therapist teaches you in the way of exercises etc. Remember they can't cure you, they can teach you how to work hard to heal yourself, but if you don't follow up the exercise routines they give you, it may take much longer to get movement back into the affected limb. If you are on pain medication, take advantage of the pain relief to do the work. There is a good feeling about participating in the healing process. I recommend it.

Sometimes my hand was in so much pain that she would massage my feet or gently rub my neck. The room where she treated me was full of plants and the smell of the oils and herbs that she uses for massage permeate her home. Marilena is a Buddhist and her home is a very peaceful and relaxing environment and it was perfect in that after each session I didn't have to travel too far to get home. By now my hand was strangely mottled and the colour of a reddish purple bruise. A friend later commented on her concerns about its appearance at this time.

> *"I was really shocked by the way it looked and how cold it was. It was so swollen and the lack of circulation made it look as though it was dying."*

Of course she didn't say that to me at the time, although I had considered it myself. Sometimes when Marilena was treating me, just the slightest touch in the 'wrong' place would send searing pain right through my hand and up my arm. She mixed up herbal tinctures which would relieve some of the nerve pain.

I have many friends, who practice meditation including Elizabeth, but I have never really got into it, so when Marilena suggested I try some pain meditation I was not really keen to start with. I thought that there was too much noise in my head. Then as time went on and I began to realise that I had nothing to lose and that I should try everything possible to alleviate the relentless pain. After the massage one night we tried it. Marilena sat in the lotus position on the floor and unfortunately because of my knee situation, I had to sit on a chair. I was beginning to feel very old. Anyway we sat quietly with our eyes closed and then she told me to imagine when I was breathing in that a white light was washing over my pain in my hand and shoulder and when I breathed out that the pain was leaving out through my fingertips in that breath.

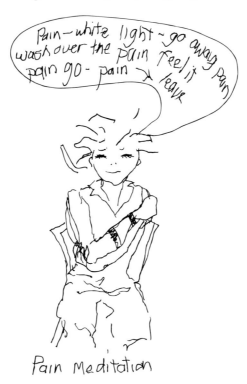

Pain Meditation

She suggested I choose a colour which represented the pain so that I could visualise it leaving my body. Now I know there are going to be some cynics among you, as indeed I was to a certain extent, but because if I want something to work, I completely put my mind to it and so really tried to imagine what she had described. What actually happened was that after a couple of minutes I burst into tears and sobbed uncontrollably. Now as my history shows, each time this has happened it has been positive and after a sobbing session I feel great relief, as I did on this occasion. Actually the notion of the meditation is not too far from the mirror theory, or indeed a version my mother's 'mind over matter' policy.

I don't know why I was so resistant to it. Marilena Hettema is a member of the National Institute of Medical Herbalists.

📖 **For futher reading on The National Institute of Medical Herbalists (NIMH) see page 205**

I had read that weight bearing exercises were important to prevent muscle atrophy. Terry had explained that it was important for me to try and use my hand to lift things.

On further reading I found that there were some weight bearing exercises for hand injuries. One article suggested improvising weights by using canned products. In the end I discovered something else which was better for me. Over the years, I have collected unusual pebbles and I thought these would make useful weights. I also realised that they would be much better if they were warm, because stone can be very cold. Since it was winter I placed the pebbles I had chosen on the radiator. I always checked to make sure they were not hot enough to burn my hand. If you keep checking them you will find that they take a long time to absorb the heat, but be cautious! During the summer if you have a window sill or somewhere where they can absorb the heat from the sun, that is also a good idea.

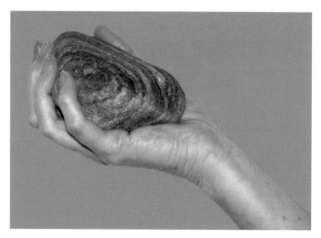

Elizabeth has arthritis in her hands and she also finds holding warm stones brings her relief. Even if you don't have your own collection of pebbles you can buy them singly at garden centres these days.

Do not use this method of exercise without consulting your Hand Therapist. It is very important that it is not done too soon after an injury as it could make things worse. After surgery it would be completely wrong. I always spoke to my Hand Therapist before doing any exercises outside of the routine they had given me to work on. Guessing is not good and can be counterproductive. Terry had agreed that it was time for me to begin weight bearing exercises.

Terry also suggested that I begin to try carrying shopping bags with my injured hand. This was less easy than the rocks and took much longer to achieve.

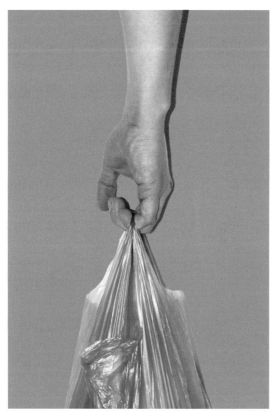

Try using day to day activities to exercise

Always consult your Occupational Therapist or physiotherapist or doctor before doing anything like this. Your break could be different to mine and this kind of thing may be good for me, but detrimental to you.

At this stage my hand was still very tight and inflexible. I would have to use the healthy hand to gently hook the handles of the plastic bag (which was resting on the floor and containing a couple of potatoes or similar) over my clawed fingers. Then I could try to lift it. This exercise could only be done for short spells as the oedema would accumulate very quickly when my hand was not elevated.

Understanding CRPS

One of the other important discoveries while surfing the net looking for an answer to the CRPS question, was that so many bloggers who have CRPS all talk about the fact that people don't understand how all encompassing and perpetual the sensations of CRPS are. It is different from anything I have ever experienced. My nose has been broken, I have had my skull fractured, a torn ligament, slipped disc etc and although certainly with the ligament and disc it was very painful, nothing compares to the range of sensations CRPS delivers. It is tugging away at you night and day. Burning, freezing, shooting, cramping contracting in such an exaggerated way that it is hard to describe to anyone else. I have tried to describe it to women by saying that it would be like being in labour for the rest of their foreseeable future at the same time as having toothache in both top and bottom jaws, but the truth is, pain is forgettable and unless you are going through it yourself, it is hard to understand.

There is a saying that if we could remember pain
most women would never have more than one child.

My friend May had an accident recently when making pancakes using a hand held food mixer. She accidentally switched it on whilst wiping the pancake mix out of the tip, with her index finger. I guarantee that anyone reading this winced at May's misfortune. For some reason we can all imagine that kind of pain, even if we have never done anything like that, but CRPS pain does not correspond to any identifiable pattern of sensations, so it remains elusive to those witnessing someone they care for who is suffering from it. As a result of all this quite often and without meaning to friends and family, and indeed the medical profession think that you are dwelling on your predicament and believe that it is 'all in the mind'. I think that it is also very difficult for them to know how to respond – I mean – what can you say?

Just a note here to say May was extremely stoical about her injury and also had to assume the 'wave position' but with one finger. So she had the appearance of someone who had just had an idea!

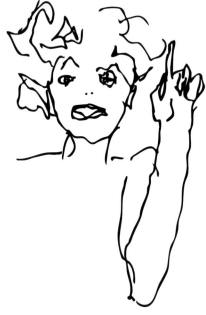

May's Finger

The level of constant pain associated with CRPS can produce deep depression in anyone experiencing it, largely because it is difficult to think about anything else and it is almost impossible to sleep – a very dangerous combination. Fatigue on its own can result in depression and in my case the thoughts that were generated in the small hours were usually pretty gloomy. I was really quite scared, but thankfully Terry and then Joseph (the Occupational Therapists) have instilled in me the importance of movement and so I had something to work on, even though at that stage there was very little movement possible. When I woke in the night I would use that time to lie there and do the hand and arm exercises and still do. I was concentrating on my posture as well, but sometimes I would find myself adopting an unusual stance, where I was trying to protect my hand and it probably looked as though I was exaggerating the pain, but as anyone with CRPS will know, a tiny bump can feel like a resounding blow, many months after the original injury. There is also that tugging feeling as though there is a string being pulled in the arm which draws the hand into a claw and it naturally moves into a position almost between the breasts. This is also a protective stance. Fighting this is a full time occupation. Try not to succumb to this position.

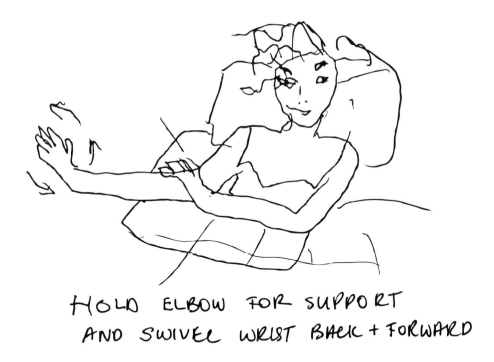

HOLD ELBOW FOR SUPPORT
AND SWIVEL WRIST BACK + FORWARD

There is an exercise which I found was useful in trying to maintain movement in my elbow as the cramp, which was perpetually there, became really unbearable if I found myself in this position for any length of time.

I found when doing most exercises at this stage that I needed to support my arm or wrist with my other hand. To attempt to do them without support was almost impossible in terms of the pain factor. As much as I wanted to resist taking too much pain medication, I have to admit that it certainly helped at night to dull down the pain a little.

I can see why anti-depressants are offered and I understand that apparently in small doses they act as pain killers, because they calm the nerves, but I am still glad I managed without them.

Overall though I think that the most important thing to realise for anyone who has a member of the family or a friend with CRPS is that the pain is all encompassing and profoundly disturbing. It is not that you can grip the location in the way you can with some pains, because the skin itself is so torturously painful and anyway the pains are like lightening passing up and down the affected limb, so most of the pain feels so deep.

I have read about some CRPS patients whose condition has spread all over their bodies. I cannot imagine the agony that they must feel.

BONES, FOOD AND THINGS

While I waited for my bone density appointment, I began to think very seriously about my diet. It is generally agreed these days that certain foods can be very beneficial, not only in sustaining good health, but in promoting the healing process.

I was now experiencing very bad circulation, aching joints and the appearance of arthritis in my index finger knuckle. I was given the number of a nutritionist who I was told was a "Top Guy". I immediately felt that this meant that he would be inaccessible unless large amounts of money were to be forked out. I was very mistaken, for instead of that, he spoke to me on the phone for a full 20 minutes. I suggested I should make an appointment to see him and he explained that he had retired to a remote part of Scotland, but didn't mind trying to help. What follows is the list of do's and don'ts that he advised. These are the things he said would be good for calcium and circulation and as anti-oxidants.

He explained that sardines have high calcium content. Fresh food is always preferable, but at that time I used the tinned ones because they were easier, since friends were helping me. They are delicious mashed up and mixed with chopped onions and chillies a squeeze of lemon and lots of black pepper. They are great like this on toast or rye biscuits.

Cut out cashews + peanuts as they leech calcium. Instead eat Brazil nuts and almonds and sesame which are full of calcium. It is an idea to grind sesame

in a coffee grinder and sprinkle it onto salads or stir it into yoghurt. Once it is ground it is easier for your system to absorb the nutrients.
If you are a coffee drinker don't have more than 2 cups per day. Preferably none at all. Coffee, he explained, also leeches calcium.

Eat lots of pineapple which has high Vitamin C content. Among other things Vitamin C apparently helps to lay down connective tissue which is involved in the healing of wounds. Vitamin C is considered an anti-oxidant and as such it is known to help eliminate free radicals which exist in our bodies as by products of pollution, alcohol and fried foods. They cause damage to the cells in the body. Blackberries and blueberries also act as anti-oxidants.

Try to sprout as many beans as you can. He told me that sprouts are fantastically good for you and contain high levels of protein and calcium.

Seaweeds are very nutritious and although not everyone likes the taste, it is really worth eating them. Add them to rice with some sesame seeds and soy sauce and bean sprouts. Plenty of Garlic purifies the blood.
Broccoli is one of the best anti-oxidants you can get. I can eat it every day. I love it with lashings of olive oil, crushed black pepper and a squeeze of lemon. Broccoli also contains high levels of Calcium, Magnesium and Vitamin C.

Herbs and spices like cloves, cumin, ginger, oregano, rosemary and thyme are rich in magnesium. Tumeric is a wonder spice and is recognised to have anti-inflammatory qualities. **Always consult your doctor before using herbs and spices if you are pregnant.**

Eat as many apples as you can. They are a powerful anti-oxidant. If possible and within your budget try to use organic ones. If not make sure to peel them. For this you will probably need help and many of the other diet suggestions may seem impossible using only one hand, but the chopping boards and other devices available from Homecraft (opposite page) make many things possible.

📖 **For Homecraft contact information see page 239**

As winter drew in and it got colder the lack of circulation in my hand became more and more of a problem. It was always a purple or reddish colour and ice cold. I know that those who have other regional pain syndromes like arthritis

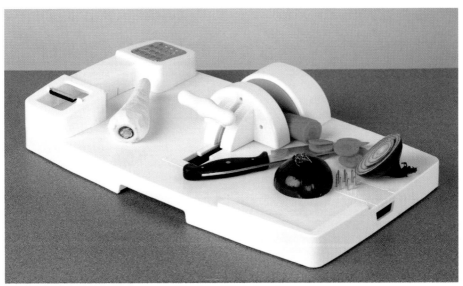

Kitchen Work Station

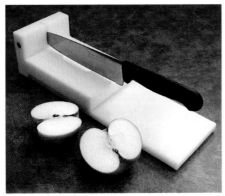

Space saver chopping board

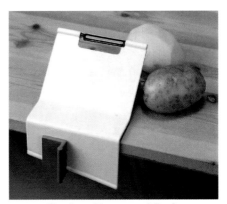

Gordon Clamp and Peeler

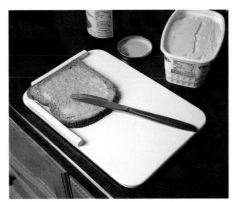

Plastic spread board

will recognise this problem. Apart from all the other weird and <u>not</u> wonderful symptoms I was experiencing, this new one was more logical and I could feel a dark ache in my bones where the fracture had taken place and in my joints which had been immobilised by the crush injury and the swelling caused by the CRPS. Having researched CRPS so much I realised, that for most, sweating and heat is one of the main symptoms. In fact during the American Civil War they referred to these sweats as 'vinegar sweats' because of the acrid odour they can sometimes give off. For me this was not the case. I had burning sensations, but my hand didn't sweat nor did it actually feel hot in the way described in many definitions. On the contrary it felt icy cold and dry even during the burning sensations. There was however an acrid odour beneath the casts in those early days of my injury.

📖 **For Causalgia CRPS and American Civil War see page 223**

I was now seeing Lizzy regularly (twice a week) for Alexander Technique and although I was still staggering with pain on some days, we were making real progress and since The Alexander Technique is so subtle I was able to relax a bit more when Lizzie gently moved my shoulder or neck. The Alexander Technique was teaching me to be continually aware of posture when I was sitting and when I walked, to be aware of not hunching my shoulders into a protective and vulnerable stance. Lizzie showed me how to carry my rucksack, how long the straps should be to eliminate further discomfort. She taught me how to sit at the computer – always squarely. Never with one leg over the other. The height that the computer should be to ensure that my neck was not under strain. Every time I left a session of Alexander Technique I felt taller and my breathing was more regular and I could really feel the difference to my whole system.

Marlilena meanwhile mixed up lotions for me and gently massaged my hands, shoulders and feet. I still couldn't lie on my front on the massage bed because my knees were so tender and my shoulder still so painful, so as usual I would receive my massage sitting in a chair. We were now making sure that both sides of my body were receiving the same care to try and encourage a connection within my whole body (as Lizzy was doing in Alexander Technique). Joseph (OT) was concerned that my fingers were not able to straighten and were still persistently trying to claw. He suggested I try to sleep in a splint to prevent them from doing so. He fashioned one for me out of the Thermoplastic.

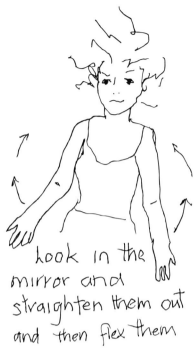

look in the
mirror and
straighten them out
and then flex them

Try to unlock injured elbow to prevent cramp

As I mentioned in Chapter Four I found that I had a tendency to draw my hand in for protection. The movement being that I bent my elbow and cradled my wrist and hand just above my waist, fingers pointing upwards between my breasts. This was comforting when there was a chance that something might bump into it, but I found it very important to counter that stance as soon as the danger had passed, otherwise my elbow would become cramped and ache. If you have this tendency while you are out, try to make sure that as soon as you get home and you feel safe, unlock your arm. Try looking in the mirror and taking note of both arms and hands and try to line them up. Look at your posture. Treat these exercises as seriously as brushing your teeth. Work on moving your hand day and night. Keep up any exercise that your Hand or Foot Therapist may give you. It might seem tedious and as though each day you have to start at the beginning, but it is so important to at least arrest the stiffness and not allow it to spread. Please keep moving and trying to use your limb!

I dreaded putting on the splint at night because it would pretty much guarantee a sleepless night and it felt regressive, although I knew that it would be beneficial in the long run and I totally trusted Joseph. Apart from being uncomfortable during the night it was excruciating when I took it off. Usually in the small hours of the morning when I craved relief. It's that feeling as though the pain has been dammed and then suddenly allowed to flow again. Terry had been right about trying very early in the treatment to get some movement in the joints. Like scar tissue, the area around each knuckle felt tight and very stuck. The overwhelming feeling of the tugging and congealing glue in my hand, elbow and arm persisted and a dark pain ran from my middle finger up through my elbow and into my shoulder and neck.

I researched more anatomical images, this time of the nerves running from the hand into the arm and shoulder. It made so much more sense that the pains were neurological.

Grays Anatomy illustrations are very clear.

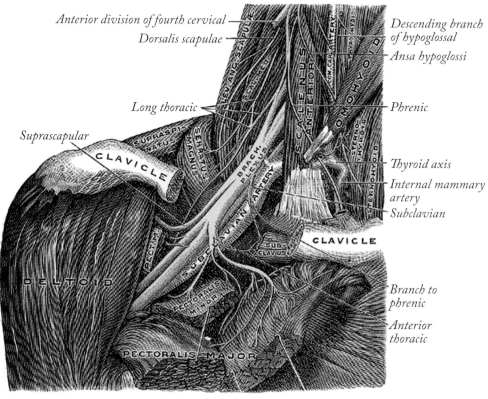

Brachial Plexus
Henry Gray 1821–1865

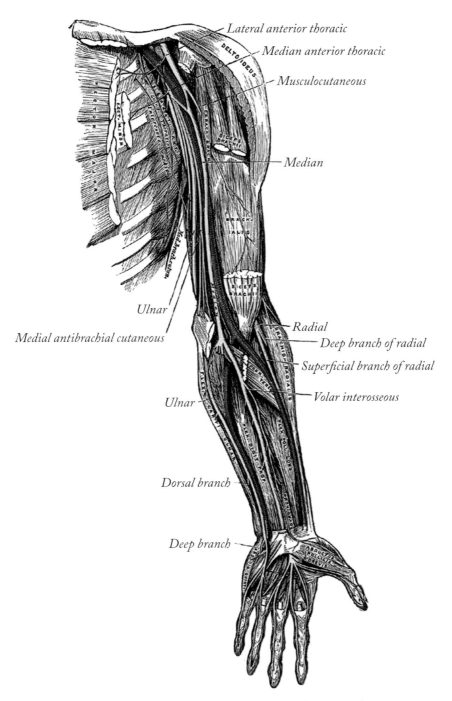

Lateral anterior thoracic

Median anterior thoracic

Musculocutaneous

Median

Ulnar

Medial antibrachial cutaneous

Radial

Deep branch of radial

Superficial branch of radial

Ulnar

Volar interosseous

Dorsal branch

Deep branch

Nerves of the Upper Extremity Grays Anatomy Fig 816
Henry Gray 1821–1865

Sometimes when I would go to have Occupational Therapy with Joseph, I would arrive in tears because either someone had bumped into me on a busy station or I'd had a bout of muscle contractions or cramps, which would literally floor me. I would arrive feeling frustrated and frightened, but a visit to that unit always cheered me up and I always left there smiling.

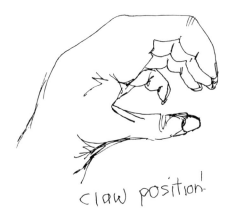

claw position!

There was a ridge in my fingernails which recorded the trauma as clearly as a geological sample records an earthquake or volcano. The ridge moved down the nail beds as they grew and Elizabeth and I watched anxiously to see if the new nail would be gnarled as had been described in some of the definitions on the web. Elizabeth was paying a lot of attention to massaging my nails and cuticles to promote circulation and thankfully although there were signs of some vertical ridging, there was no deformity. Much later Joseph admitted that he had also been slightly apprehensive about the possible health of the new nail as we had watched that ridge descend. Another milestone to be celebrated.

THINGS THAT JANGLE NERVES

I would go down on weekends to visit Elizabeth and Jeff and Elizabeth would 'massage' my hand at least twice a day. She was still encouraging me to access any treatments which might be beneficial and constantly assured me that she would fund any expenses. It is important to note this, because I believe that without that financial help, to keep up my rigorous regime, I would probably have become a long term burden to the NHS. Although there is some recognition these days that things like Acupuncture, Alexander, Acupressure and massage are beneficial, it is extremely difficult to access them. Some may think that "I would have got better in due course" but I know how hard it has been to keep up the exercises and how much work others have put into my recovery. Even though at the time of writing this, it is almost two years ago that the accident happened, I still have to keep up the exercises to stop my hand feeling rigid, particularly in damp weather conditions.

Often during that period Elizabeth would come up to London for the sole purpose of massaging my hand. I know that this unconditional expression of love from her was also so important in my healing. I could see at times in spite of the fact that she was tired, she forced herself to do it and insisted even when the pain was so bad that I tried to resist. She knew we had to keep it moving and I will be eternally grateful to her. She is still as attentive to my hand as ever.

Below is a photograph of the restriction resulting from my crush injury.

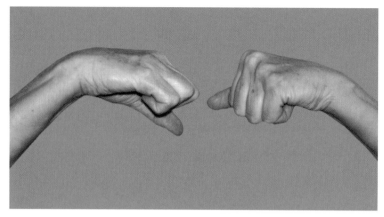

My right hand cannot make a fist. The MCP Joints (The Big Knuckles) are damaged.
Photograph taken 2010.

As I have mentioned Elizabeth experiences arthritis in her hands and has managed to keep it at bay with diet, massage, herbs and various alternative treatments over the years. She told me that the massaging of my hands was therapeutic for hers. I liked the dynamic of that.

Christmas came and went and my hand and shoulder remained in an agonising state in spite of Elizabeth's constant attention and all the other therapies. I know that they were all contributing to the reduction of oedema, to circulation and to movement, which would be invaluable in the long term, but the CRPS was taking a firm grip, **literally**! I was now experiencing crippling contractions and spasms. Because of the winter weather, my hand became somewhat more swollen and rigid. The skin was thin, tight and shiny and ranged in colour from purple to blue to mottled grey. I was once again unable to move my wrist freely and I had to constantly wear an oedema glove to try to control the swelling. The shoulder was so painful that even doing small things like zipping my trousers was near impossible and made me weep. I had had to give up the days I loved to spend in Shal's garden because I couldn't really do much; I was so dogged with spasms of such paralyzing pain. It is a characteristic of CRPS that there will be fluctuations in the intensity of the symptoms which often are not determined by any particular stimulus or activity. I did continue the mirror work though and it continued to give temporary pain relief and helped me perform the movement exercises. It also re-enforced for me the importance of viewing my injured hand in a positive way. In retrospect I regret that I did not use the mirror therapy as often as I could have during this period. I think that it needs to be done very regularly for the best results.

It was now three months since my request for a bone density test and I still didn't have an appointment. I was fearful that my bones might be in the process of atrophying because of the stiffness and lack of movement in my knuckles. Joseph (OT) tried to help me access some physiotherapy for my shoulder, but we ran into a dead end. We meanwhile continued working on trying to prevent my hand from stiffening and to promote circulation as much as possible. Joseph really was an enormous support during those bleak months. His gentle encouragement and genuine interest in what was happening to me was so important. The wax bath was always something I looked forward to, it seemed to thaw my hand for short periods which gave relief from the cramps, but on the whole I think that this was the worst period for me.

The GP who I had been seeing was away on leave and I got the impression from the person standing in for him, that the fact I was already having Occupational Therapy for my hand made it less likely that I would be able to be referred for physiotherapy for my shoulder as well. She didn't say it in so many words, but when I asked for the referral she looked at my notes and said impatiently "But you are already having Occupational Therapy." When my frustration resulted in tears, she again looked at my notes and asked me if I had been taking the anti-depressants which I had been prescribed. I had to reply that I was not as depressed about the CRPS as I was about trying to access treatment which might prevent me becoming an unnecessary statistic on incapacity benefit. She seemed irritated and said that the anti-depressants at low dosage help with pain. I replied that I was not keen on taking anti-depressants.

In retrospect, if at that time anyone had carefully explained to me the thinking behind how anti-depressants can sometimes be helpful with nerve pain I might have tried them, because I can see the sense in it. I am however aware of so many people who have been prescribed anti-depressants as a panacea for anything that might cause anxiety that I was very resistant and scared that they would just mask the symptoms and I would be in more danger. Nobody had actually checked my shoulder and I still think it is so important to have some sort of diagnosis before you begin to take medication. It also occurred to me that there was a strong possibility that the GPs don't really know how Occupational Therapy or Physiotherapy work and that each part is treated in isolation, so although I was receiving Occupational Therapy in a Hand Unit, my elbow and shoulder remained unattended.

Thankfully Joseph showed concern and has always treated me with care physically and psychologically because at times I found some of the attitudes towards me and this horrible condition nothing short of callous. I'm no wimp but it sometimes wore me down so I can't imagine how others who have less support than me manage to cope with the attitude of some in the Health Service Industry who seem oblivious to the suffering of their patients. Perhaps the system has become so fragmented that it is not always possible for health-care professionals to see the full picture.

📖 **For details on The Patients Association see page 209**

In due course I finally received a notification from the Osteoporosis Scanning Unit giving me a date for my bone density scan. I attended and found the department really well run and pleasant and efficient. The results, I was told, would be sent back to my GP within 10 days, but were usually received within one week.

It was now the middle of winter and the cold and damp were playing havoc with my injured joints. Once when the pain was so overwhelming that I was huddled on the floor near my fridge, I decided to phone Demian and ask him if he had any tips. His tip was quite unexpected and although I couldn't put it into practice at that moment, I realised how valuable and far reaching the notion of it was in the long term for my condition. At the time just talking to someone who understood the nature of nerve pain helped me to cope.

Demian's Tip: As soon as possible, go and listen to live classical music. Now I know that this will seem completely bonkers at first, but he explained that the resonance of the music calms the nerves and since CRPS is the result of damaged nerves, it made perfect sense. I thought back to the day at the fracture clinic when the TV was blasting out a treble sound of mindless cartoons in the background, and how it wound me up. I thought then that I was probably just a 'grumpy old woman' but I now realised that the frequency and resonance was not conducive to the calming of nerves. I made a note to be aware of sounds and whether they triggered nerve pain. "Think of a fingernail scratching on a blackboard." I never actually made it to a live concert but began listening to more classical music when I was at home. Steer clear of anything used on call centre telephone queues!

Taiwan and Ko Medicine

During my research on the web, I had found a treatment called Collateral Meridian Therapy – CMT. It particularly caught my eye because there was a testimonial from a patient who had been suffering with CRPS in his foot. After receiving the CMT Treatment he described the release from the tugging, heavy, gummed up feeling he had been experiencing.

That gummed up feeling is one of the most overriding and constant sensations of the syndrome. I think that putting aside the severe pain this is one of the most worrying symptoms of CRPS.

After a while it becomes so obvious that the pain is related to the nerves, but the gumming up is more of a physical manifestation, and unlike the cramps and muscle spasms it is not sporadic and remains constant. It feels literally as though the limb is full of congealing glue, becoming heavier and heavier as it congeals. It is a very frightening experience because it is as if slowly, but surely, your limb is losing its life.

The testimonial excited me so much because that and many other sensations he described corresponded exactly to the symptoms I was experiencing. I suddenly felt hopeful and I yearned for that release. In fact that had been a major motivation to continue the exercises in the hope that one day my wrist would just click and that horrible heavy sensation would be gone. I was fascinated by the copies of the patient's bone scans.

Dr. Ko who developed Ko Medicine works through a company called **Enrac** who are based in Taiwan. Dr. Ko is Taiwanese and spent the last thirty years trying to find ways of reducing pain without resorting to vast prescriptions of pain killers and anti-depressants.

📖 **For further reading on Dr. Ko see pages 212 and 237**

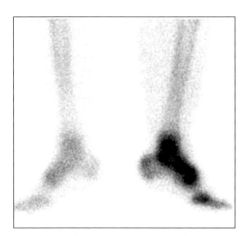 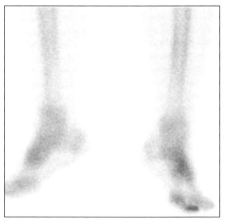

Three phase bone scans of a CRPS patient before (left) and after (right) CMT

I contacted an Enrac representative who was in the US, a Shang Ko. (not related to the Dr. Ko who developed Enrac CMT) I had long discussions with him on email. He was very supportive and explained that I could contact the Painless Ginza Clinic in Japan where Dr. Ko practises CMT. He also told me that unfortunately there were very long waiting times for CMT treatment in Japan, but that I might be able to access some treatment in Taipei where most of the hospitals are beginning to use Ko Medicine (Enrac CMT) as treatment for chronic pain. Elizabeth and I discussed how I could get there to receive the treatment.

I telephoned the Taiwanese offices of Enrac and they immediately organised for me to have some treatment in Taiwan. It was so marvellous, in spite of the slight difficulties arising out of the language differences to be able to talk about CRPS with people who were very familiar with it.
I hurriedly arranged a flight and phoned the bone density clinic to make sure my results had in fact been sent to my GP. I needed a copy of them that I could

take with me to Taiwan. I had also received notification that I had an appointment at a Pain Clinic on that Friday. This was the referral which was made for me at the appointment where my 'frozen shoulder' had been diagnosed on that awful day at the fracture clinic. I was very pleased and hopeful that who-ever I was going to see at the pain clinic would be more familiar with CRPS and therefore more interested than the GP or those at the very busy fracture clinic. This was on a Friday and I was booked to leave on the Sunday. I thought it important to take the bone density results with me to that meeting as well.

To cut a long boring story short I was told at the GP Surgery that my results had not been received. On my insistence that the Imaging Department had assured me that they had been sent and would have arrived there the previous Tuesday, they were grudgingly found but I was told that I couldn't access them because the doctor had not seen them. They had been there for three days and although I had written a letter requesting them as soon as possible, this had been ignored. Unfortunately as in many cases like this one, your fate can rest in the hands of a receptionist wielding power over people at their most vulnerable. The person in question said that the pain clinic could fax a request through for the results, but I knew how short these appointments were and how inefficient the GP's filing system appeared to be, so I decided to give up the idea of taking it to the pain clinic, but I did want to have a copy to take to Taiwan.

When you ask for a referral or are told that you have been given one, ask how long you should expect to wait. If you have waited an unreasonable amount of time, write a polite letter confirming what you were told at your appointment. This is necessary because sometimes because of computer systems or whatever, your referral could get lost. **Don't sit waiting for months to find out you are not even in the queue!** It is your right to question what is happening. Mostly you will receive an appointment very quickly after writing.

When I said that I was going abroad for some treatment and that I needed the results, I was told to call back and if the doctor had time (*he was very busy with his patients!*) they would get him to look at the results and then I would be able to collect them. I tried calling but was told he had not looked at them and so I accepted that I would not be taking them with me to Taiwan either. I would like to point out here that it took four months for me to get an appointment from the time I asked the GP, even though I was told at the

Imaging Department that it was unheard of to take longer than three weeks. It took one week to get the results sent to the surgery and after four days of them having arrived, I was still prevented from accessing them.

The visit to the pain clinic was not awful and I didn't have to wait. I found the doctor interested and empathic. I was still in some considerable pain, but the swelling was much less than is normally associated with CRPS at this stage (7 months) because of all the treatments I have already described. My three injured fingers however were still stuck tightly together and from the knuckle joint went rigidly straight out with the tips of the fingers trying to claw. It was like being in a perpetual cramp and my thumb ached. The clawing sensation is very strong, so the fact that I physically could not make a fist added to this conflict and cramped horribly.

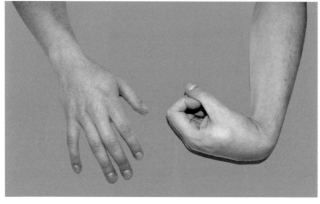

In the long term CRPS can result in the hand drawing inwards and locking in that position (this is an example of the stance and is not a picture of CRPS)

The doctor at the Pain Clinic listened with interest to my account of all the things I had been doing to try and recover and was equally as interested in my imminent journey to Taiwan and the proposed treatment there. He asked me what I had hoped to find at the pain clinic since I had been fairly successful on the route I had chosen. I explained that I had been waiting for an appointment for four months and that I liked to keep all appointments because I was so determined to get better and that I had thought that this would be a place where CRPS was known and maybe understood. I also explained that I had hoped that they might be able to help me access Acupuncture etc. without having to pay private fees. He looked doubtful and so I asked him what in fact he would be able to offer and his reply was that unfortunately the support would be more in the way of medication than anything else.

I need to point out again here that I had read a lot of blog sites and many experiencing CRPS described the adverse effects of multiple combinations of pain medications taken in the long term. Some even talked of ulcerated stomachs, so I was keen not to become someone who was dependent on that kind of treatment.

It was a cold, grey day and although I had been trying to keep my spirits up in spite of the shooting pains and ache in my elbow, I felt I had just reached a sort of dead end and I sat on the pavement in an alley and wept with frustration again. I was still very aware of how fortunate I was that I had other options, even if they took me to the other side of the world – literally!

I flew out of Heathrow for Taiwan in February on what some perceived as my rather desperate adventure. As usual Elizabeth had focussed on how to alleviate as much pain as possible on the long journey and gave me a small 'squishy' micro bead support cushion that could fit into my hand luggage. These cushions really are very good for travel purposes and mould into a supportive shape. This one was in a fine stretchy fabric, allowing it to adapt its shape to the required contour. Micro bead cushions are much like a normal bean bag, but instead of beans they are stuffed with beads probably somewhere between the size of a mustard seed and a poppy seed. They are very lightweight. Elizabeth's one worked really well both as a soft support for my elbow on the hard seat rest and at times moulded into my neck. I had a window seat so that my hand was out of harm's way and my journey was more bearable than I had anticipated although the cabin pressure did contribute to the swelling in my hand.

Quite a few of my friends had been alarmed that I would head off into the unknown to be treated. It was probably a measure of the level of my pain and frustration at my experiences at times in the NHS; feeling like a criminal or trouble maker in some quarters when I expressed any interest or knowledge of what was happening in my body. I actually felt much less afraid of this journey than I did of going to the fracture clinic in London. The holistic approach appealed to me. The idea that, like Acupuncture the focus of the healing was centred in certain meridians – lines of life force (if you like) which are located close to the skeleton. I particularly liked the idea that my hand was not going to be treated in isolation to the rest of my body. Joseph, like the Doctor at the Pain Clinic was interested in the Taiwanese treatments.

As I have mentioned before, often in my research about CRPS I found it well understood that a multidisciplinary approach is the best, so in a way that was what was happening with me. Usually, a multidisciplinary approach includes a fair amount of medication and very often nerve blockers or invasive treatments along-side hands on therapies and psychological support. My multidisciplinary approach didn't include much in the way of medication, thankfully.

The travel agent had found me a good hotel in the centre of Taipei, but I had opted to have my treatment in Tao Yuan which is about a 40 minute train ride from Taipei. Let me explain. Anyone with CRPS will testify that no matter what you do, the pain is electrifying and my way of dealing with it was to keep trying to do things, to keep walking, moving and trying to keep my mind busy, and my circulation going, so the train trips to Tao Yuan and back were interesting and useful in that respect. I also think that being out and about helps to avoid succumbing to depression. You are in pain anyway and it doesn't really help to just stay indoors and be fearful. Also if you keep moving at least the tiredness you feel at the end of the day is more physical fatigue and not just emotional fatigue and anxiety which can hinder sleep even more.

On my first morning David (The Taiwanese Enrac interpreter) arrived at the hotel to accompany me to my meeting with a Dr. Wang in Tao Yuan. David had lived in America for most of his childhood and into his twenties so communication was easy. I was not really sure whether I would have treatment that day or just a consultation. Anyway we took the train to a hospital in Tao Yuan where Dr. Wang (who also speaks fluent English) greeted me warmly and conducted a very comprehensive examination and questionnaire about my condition. As you will now know I travel everywhere with a full file including copies of x rays, doctors letters etc., so after studying the file and photocopying all this for her records, Dr. Wang began to write a prescription of meridian points for my treatment. She told me that there were two options for the treatment. Acupressure with acu sticks which would be pushed firmly down on the pressure points by herself and three other technicians. This meant at least 5–6 points being pushed down for 2 minutes for each prescribed action. The other alternative was that they could use a sort of tens machine on the same points. I asked what the difference would be and she explained that it would be more painful with the acu sticks, but much more effective. Since I knew I was only here for a short time I opted for the acu sticks treatment.

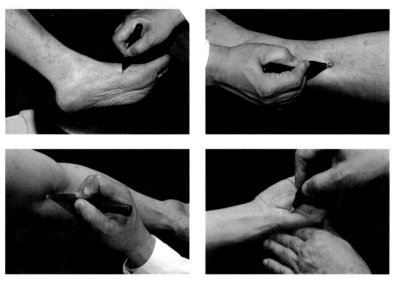

Pictures from Enrac CMT Manual of Patient having CMT

Nothing could have prepared me for the pain that followed, but at least I could understand what they were doing. They were trying to redirect the pain into another meridian where it would eventually dissipate. I imagined this would allow the injury to heal without the barrage of pain that was being directed to it endlessly by the scrambled neurological messages.

Since my treatment in February 2008 Enrac have introduced an E System which minimises the pain of the procedure. I am glad about this because it makes CMT easier for me to recommend. However it was not the treatment I was given, so I can only describe my own experience. No matter how painful the treatment was at the time, I would do it all again, because it worked! It took away enough of the CRPS pain for me to see a light at the end of the tunnel. It gave me hope to add to Elizabeth's and my dogged determination to find a way to for me to get better.

I have to say I was pretty exhausted and shaken going back on the train with David, but he was kind and funny and we chatted and he did manage to make me giggle on the way back to Taipei. That night for the first time in nearly eight months, with the exception of my Acupuncture nights, I slept soundly through till morning. Something had shifted and I was keen to see the results of more treatment.

📖 For details on Enrac and CMT see page 212

After two days I went again for treatment with Dr. Wang in Tao Yuan and this time the pain in my elbow disappeared completely. I could feel that as I dressed to leave the hospital.

Dr. Wang had told me that I could have my third treatment in Taipei on the Sunday as she would be there attending a conference where I would be able to meet Dr. Ko. who is the person who developed CMT.

📖 For historical reference on CMT see page 237

Having had the two sessions with Dr. Wang and her assistants, I felt a little weak at the prospect of more of the painful treatment, but the results were so astounding that I was absolutely determined to carry on. The searing pain that I had worn like a glove on my hand was not nearly as extreme as it had been and the skin on my hand did not burn so intensely. The cold dark pain in my elbow had completely gone. The relief in my elbow had been so absolute and so fast that I was hopeful that the next session would relieve the paralyzing pain in my shoulder, and the deep pains and contractions in my hand which were still dogging me.

I decided to make the most of my time in Taipei so I woke up on the Sunday morning which was beautiful and sunny and after breakfast took the hotel courtesy bus to Taipei Main Station. Then I walked the extra six blocks which took me through Peace Park. Although I know the Park was named for historical reasons, it was well named for me on that day because there were hundreds of little birds feeding on the lawns and a general ambiance of their chirping, which was not shrill but melodic and relaxing. Couples and families were walking about quietly chatting. It definitely felt very peaceful and calmed my perpetually jangled nerves. There were market stalls selling sweets and nuts and ground black sesame. I bought a bag of the sesame to sprinkle on my

Tofu breakfast. Both tofu and sesame (particularly black sesame) are high in calcium content and very beneficial for healthy bones.

When I arrived at the Enrac Centre I was shown to a conference hall where Dr. Ko (who I recognised from the photograph I had seen on the web) was enthusiastically lecturing to an audience of about 20–30 people. Sofi who had been my contact at Enrac ushered me into the hall and straight to the front urging me to talk about my condition and about whether the treatments had relieved me of any pain.

At first I felt a little anxious about this and then decided that since I had taught English as a foreign language it wouldn't be the first time that I had stood in front of a room full of people who didn't speak English. My stage fright was short lived and so was my speech and then I was thankfully shown to a room where I would have some treatment with Dr. Wang after which we would join the others for an early lunch and then the conference would continue.

Dr. Wang took me through to large room where Dr. Ko was diagnosing a patient while a group from the conference observed. When he was finished Dr. Wang introduced us and showed Dr. Ko my x ray. He took my hand in his and studied it, all the while explaining in Chinese to his colleagues his prognosis, while Dr. Wang translated for me. Dr. Ko suggested I attend the Clinic in Tao Yuan a couple of days later where he would make his own assessment and administer more treatment. I felt utterly comfortable with Dr. Ko. He was full of confidence and excitement having had positive proof in thousands of cases that the Collateral Meridian Therapy was able to deliver instant pain relief. However Dr. Wang did tell me that Dr. Ko had said that it would take more time in my case because of the severity of the CRPS.

I was also introduced to a charming man who I was told by Dr. Wang was an eminent orthopaedic surgeon in Taipei, a Dr. Au who also spoke fluent English. I expressed my fears about bone atrophy and arthritis and he listened carefully and assured me that as long as I had no record of osteoporosis and if I kept moving my limb as much as possible I could prevent any of these things happening. He explained that Dr. Ko and Collateral Meridian Therapy were held in very high regard in Taiwan where CMT was being introduced into hospitals to help those experiencing intractable pain. He told me how sports injuries were being successfully treated and how CMT was becoming very popular in that field because it enabled patients to recover much more quickly once the pain was eliminated.

We went back into the hall and I sat with Dr. Wang near the back and was given an anatomical doll displaying the CMT meridian lines. These, by the way are not the same meridians used in Acupuncture. I was also given an atlas of the pressure points to look at. I found everyone very warm and attentive.

Dr. Ko was using a projection of the meridians and began the lecture, pointing to certain lines and enthusiastically explaining to his colleagues the miracle of the CMT technique. Dr. Ko spoke Traditional Chinese (Mandarin) with a gentle tone and was completely consumed with his findings and his quest to find a route to absolute pain relief. His excitement at being able to share his extraordinary findings with others in the medical profession was obvious. At a certain point the Orthopaedic surgeon who I had talked to at lunch (Dr. Au) came through the hall and indicated that he would like to speak to me outside the room. He suggested that since it was obvious I was hungry to glean as much as I could from the lecture, and since I didn't understand Mandarin, I could make use of the resonance of Dr. Ko's voice and try to allow it to calm my damaged nerves. He suggested I concentrate on the voice and allow it to sweep through my body, like Marilena's meditation. I was really excited by the suggestion, which confirmed what Demian had told me about the resonance in classical music being something which had helped him with nerve pain, but more so that someone in this high position had taken the time to come over and say that to me. It's so obvious, that gentle sounds are soothing for nerves and Dr. Ko's voice definitely had a soothing quality to it added to the fact that what he was describing was something healing.

I think it is important to acknowledge here that there are so many layers of pain with CRPS that the fact that I felt such overwhelming relief after each CMT Treatment did not mean that the overall pain had gone. It just took away some of those layers. I was still experiencing abnormal levels of pain brought about by the CRPS. I had to be aware that as with all the other treatments, I needed to keep up the CMT if I was going to achieve any success at beating the syndrome.

There was an air of excitement by everyone at the conference. Here at last was a treatment for intractable pain which had so eluded all of them for so long. I was pleased to have been there to witness their enthusiasm and to give my account of the pain relief after my treatment with CMT.

The following week I was treated by Dr. Ko and although the treatment was very painful, the relief afterwards was so noticeable that I was again prepared to have as many treatments as I needed.

Dr. Ko told me through an interpreter that his prognosis was that I would need at least nine months of treatment, since the CRPS appeared to be severe and treatments should be spaced to give time between each one; as is the case with most therapeutic work. Now to ward off any cynics, most treatments for total recovery of the sort of crush injury I had would take that kind of time without CRPS. So far in the West I had not heard much in the way of any specific treatment which claimed to be able to entirely conquer the dogged effects of CRPS. When I asked at Enrac about what percentage of people with CRPS were completely cured, by the CMT I was told roughly 70% to 80%.

Of course my mind went immediately to how I would be able to manage to get back to Taiwan and stay for the nine months. I think that only someone with CRPS would understand that finding relief from the pain is so rare that if you feel there is a chance, it is to be embraced wholeheartedly. The notion of being away from home for such a long period of time paled in comparison to having to endure the levels of pain CRPS delivers on a minute to minute basis. I still wore the oedema glove during the day and slept most of the night in Joseph's splint.

Whatever treatments you have, nothing is going to simply deliver movement and circulation into an injured limb. That is your responsibility. What is on offer with Enrac CMT, is pain relief. Pain is the reason that we might be afraid to do exercises or try to use our hand or foot. A constant dedication to movement is the most important recovery tool you have and it is free. Everything that I have read or learnt during my last two years has convinced me of this, but if I had needed confirmation it came towards the end of my stay in Taiwan. I asked David if he, as an interpreter, had ever been present when a patient with CRPS had been told that they could not be treated by CMT, "Oh Yes" was his stark reply "sometimes it is too late if the arm or leg is too stiff from no movement for a long time."

My stay was drawing to a close when Dr. Wang told me that she and her colleagues felt that the ailment in my shoulder was not 'Frozen Shoulder', because they had treated it and that usually a frozen shoulder would respond to 2–3 treatments, whereas mine was still very painful. She suggested I have it checked on my return to London. I resolved to try and arrange an MRI scan.

I was truly sorry to leave Taipei. I had arrived in so much pain, but it had now been reduced by about 40%. Believe me this is quite significant with CRPS and especially in such a short time. My elbow no longer throbbed with the dark pain. I knew quite well though, that the condition was still very strong in my hand and my shoulder remained stiff and painful, and that I required long term treatment to conquer this horrible affliction.

I was not only sorry to leave because of the pain relief I had been receiving, it was the Taiwanese people I had met who had been so amazing and I will always remember them with the utmost affection.

This was now February over six months since the accident.

BACK IN UK,
MRI AND MIRROR BOX

The weekend of my return Mimi drove me down to Elizabeth and Jeff's house. Elizabeth had kept up a daily contact via email while I was in Taipei. It was much appreciated because sometimes after the treatment I was weepy as it was so traumatic. I was really looking forward to seeing her to show her the improvements. It was an emotional meeting as she noted that the pain had gone out of my eyes and face and we clung to each other, both holding back the tears. Elizabeth had been so intimately a part of my experience and as soon as we sat down at the table she took my hand in hers and examined it and rubbed oil into it and resumed her extraordinary massage.

For the next couple of months I continued my Alexander, massage by Elizabeth and Marilena and Occupational Therapy with Joseph. All of whom marvelled at the positive results from my trip to Taipei. I was very keen to return to Taipei and have the nine months of treatment prescribed by Dr. Ko. At this point some other friends of mine had heard about my situation and had generously written a cheque for me which would cover a considerable amount of therapy and which could make Taiwan possible. I was overwhelmed by their generosity and grateful that Elizabeth would be relieved of the costs. That same week another friend came forward and also contributed, so I now found myself in the fortunate position of being able once again to pursue any route I chose to try and find relief from the ghastly CRPS. I couldn't believe how lucky I was.

I continued doing mirror work, but found that the mirror box that Vic had made for me was quite big and took up a large space on the kitchen table. I decided to try and design one that I could fold away when I was finished because this one was beginning to take the role of another piece of furniture. Books accumulated on top of it and I would store all my lotions and therapy balls etc. inside it. It was no longer an easy exercise to start using it and I would decide to do mirror work and then look at how much stuff needed to be moved out of the way before I started and I would put it off. I began work on trying to design one that would be big enough to facilitate global exercises, (sweeping wrist movements and turning of hands without restrictions) but light enough for me to erect and to fold away with one hand. A friend told me about someone who could make it for me and so having come up with the design I sent it off to him and after a considerable amount of design problems I ended up with one that was really good and easy to manage.

At this point armed with my friends' generous funding, I decided to try and get a referral for an MRI scan for my shoulder. I knew that it would be a useless exercise approaching my GP, but now I had the opportunity to pay for one, I made an appointment to see the Consultant at the private clinic and she referred me immediately to the MRI unit upstairs. Privately MRI scans can cost between £700 – £1000 including an appointment on each side for the referral and then the reading of the results. The scans are essential to be able to see tissue damage and pretty much everything that is going on in the area of the injury. So I felt extremely privileged to be able to have one.
I wished though that I had done a bit of research about MRI's because it would have been an idea to practise shallow breathing. For those who have not had an MRI scan, it involves lying on your back and being drawn into a tunnel, where you have to lie very still while the multi resonance equipment records a sort of 3D image of your injury. It is so delicate that any movement can blur the image. You are given headphones because for some reason the process involves very loud banging sounds (like an incessant drum beat or someone running up or down metal stairs with cast iron shoes).

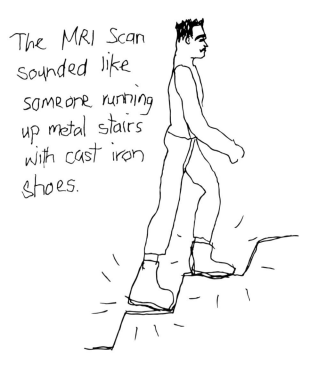

The MRI Scan sounded like someone running up metal stairs with cast iron shoes.

Anyway this all takes a long time – 40 minutes to an hour. It is a brilliant diagnostic tool and not easy to acquire so when I found myself in the tunnel, I was irritated that I was panicking a little and my breathing became erratic and so I was moving and obstructing the process. The technician assured me through the headphones that it was very common and that I should just try to relax and hold as still as I possibly could. This was when I realised that some practice in shallow breathing might have been beneficial before the scan.

If you are referred for an MRI or any other scan take time to find out what it means and do practice breathing. It will really help to prepare you for the process. At least with the information these scans provide there is less room for mistaken diagnosis.

The Consultant had explained that if there was no real problem, she would be able to give me the results of the scan but if there were problems I would have to be referred to a Shoulder Specialist who would be able to answer any questions and give me a comprehensive breakdown of the scan's findings. I was fairly convinced that there were some problems and so she referred me then and there to a Shoulder Specialist in the same hospital.

I felt very upbeat after the appointment with the shoulder specialist because he had been so interested in the various therapies I had opted for. After perusing my file, which of course I had brought with me to the appointment, he asked me to stand up and led me through various movements, some of which were very painful. He was very encouraging about the range of movements that I was able to achieve. They were apparently usually far more limited with my condition, which turned out not to be Frozen Shoulder but Subacromial Bursitis.

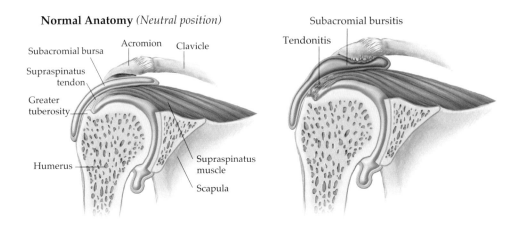

In spite of the incorrect diagnosis, the therapies that I had chosen to follow did nothing to make the situation worse. On the contrary, the Alexander Technique which concentrates largely on posture had most certainly prevented habitual protective stances that in a very short time can exaggerate the restrictions in movement already present as a result of the condition. The array of pillows that I used supported my shoulder joint when I slept, so it took any pressure or unnecessary tension on the injury. I felt very encouraged and gratified that I was heading in the right direction. I asked the Specialist about what treatment he would offer and he said that there were three options:

1. Surgery – To go in and scrape away the calcified matter (Bone spurs). Neither he nor I were in the slightest bit keen on that as a course of action.

II. A cortisone injection that would be administered with a local anaesthetic (which itself can be painful). This method is reputed to bring instant relief, thereby facilitating less painful movement which is always beneficial. I asked if it would wear off and he answered that in most cases it wears off in a few months and has to be redone. We were both in agreement that we didn't like that idea.

III. His third option, since I was not adverse to a little discomfort in the ultimate search for long term recovery, was that I continue with the Alexander Technique, Acupuncture and massage in the treatment of my shoulder and if the condition continued and remained painful after a few months that I should return.

I was really comforted by what he had said and had the distinct impression that it was not just good bedside manner, but real interest that he had shown in the various treatments I had been having. All of the treatments were playing their part in a slow and steady recovery, but my shoulder movement was very restricted and painful and I was still encountering the shooting pains and muscle contractions of the CRPS.

Now I had actually been diagnosed, I felt confident that I could go ahead and try to get my shoulder better. I was so relieved that it was not the CRPS that had moved, which is quite common. It was gratifying to encounter someone apart from the OTs and the Consultant who showed that kind of genuine interest during those painful and frightening times. One of the better encounters in mainstream medicine, it counterbalanced the disinterest shown by some others and restored my trust in the medical profession. I did though think how extraordinary it was that the Taiwanese had been able to say with some certainty that is was definitely not frozen shoulder without an MRI scan.

I made some new appointments with Dr. Zhu for more Acupuncture and continued weekly Alexander Technique with Lizzie.

My sessions with both of them were so important in helping to centre me during my experience of CRPS. They were times where, because of the nature of the treatment, you have to lie very quietly and this in itself has a calming effect on the nerves. See nerves following two pages.

In all of these sessions though I had to have support to my shoulder which was firmly locked, preventing a lot of movement and if when lying on my back it was not supported it would feel as though it was being torn apart.

Spinal Nerves

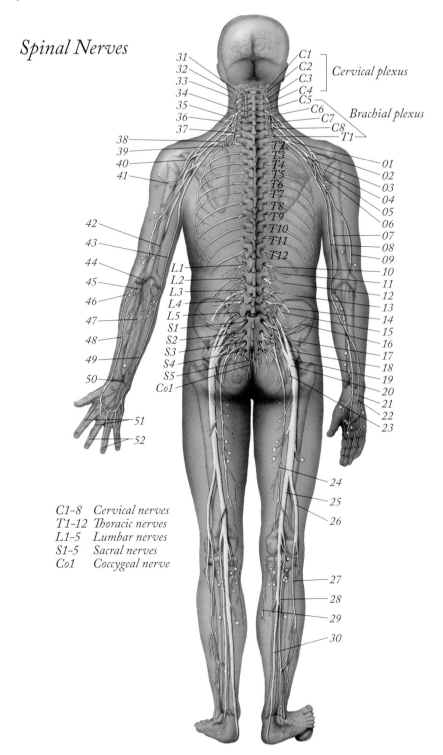

C1
C2
C3 } Cervical plexus
C4
C5
C6
C7
C8
T1

Brachial plexus

31
32
33
34
35
36
37
38
39
40
41

T2
T3
T4
T5
T6
T7
T8
T9
T10
T11
T12

01
02
03
04
05
06
07
08
09
10
11
12
13
14
15
16
17
18
19
20
21
22
23

42
43
44
45
46
47
48
49
50

L1
L2
L3
L4
L5
S1
S2
S3
S4
S5
Co1

51
52

24
25
26

27
28
29
30

C1–8 Cervical nerves
T1–12 Thoracic nerves
L1–5 Lumbar nerves
S1–5 Sacral nerves
Co1 Coccygeal nerve

© 2009 Wolters Kluwer Health | Lippincott Williams and Wilkins

01. *Posterior cord of brachial plexus – C5, C6, C7, C8, T1*
02. *Lateral cord of brachial plexus – C5, C6, C7*
03. *Medial cord of brachial plexus – C8, T1*
04. *Musculocutaneous nerve – C5, C6, C7*
05. *Axillary nerve – C5, C6*
06. *Median nerve – C5, C6, C7, C8, T1*
07. *Median nerve*
08. *Ulnar nerve – C7, C8, T1*
09. *Radial nerve – C5, C6, C7, C8, T1*
10. *Iliohypogastric nerve – T12, L1*
11. *Ilioinguinal nerve – L1*
12. *Genitofemoral nerve – L1, L2*
13. *Lateral femoral cutaneous nerve – L2, L3*
14. *Femoral nerve – L2, L3, L4*
15. *Obdurator nerve – L2, L3, L4*
16. *Superior gluteal nerve – L4, L5, S1*
17. *Inferior gluteal nerve – L5, S1, S2*
18. *Sciatic nerve – L4, L5, S1, S2, S3*
19. *Common peroneal nerve (Posterior division of ventral rami) – L4, L5, S1, S2*
20. *Tibial nerve (Anterior division of ventral rami) – L4, L5, S1, S2, S3*
21. *Median nerve*
22. *Ulnar nerve*
23. *Pudendal nerve – S2, S3, S4*
24. *Posterior femoral cutaneous nerve – S1, S2, S3*
25. *Tibial nerve – L4, L5, S1, S2, S3*
26. *Common peroneal nerve – L4, L5, S1, S2*
27. *Lateral sural cutaneous nerve – L2, L3*
28. *Medial sural cutaneous nerve*
29. *Saphenous nerve*
30. *Tibial nerve – L4, L5, S1, S2, S3*
31. *Minor occiptal nerve*
32. *Great auricular nerve*
33. *Transverse cervical nerve*
34. *Supraclavicular nerve*
35. *Dorsal scapular nerve*
36. *Suprascapular nerve*
37. *Long thoracic nerve – C5, C6, C7*
38. *Medial pectoral nerve – C8, T1*
39. *Medial cutaneous nerve of arm and forearm*
40. *Musculocutaneous nerve – C5, C6, C7*
41. *Axillary nerve – C5, C6*
42. *Median nerve*
43. *Ulnar nerve*
44. *Radial nerve – C5, C6, C7, C8, T1*
45. *Deep branch of radial nerve*
46. *Lateral cutaneous nerve of forearm*
47. *Posterior interosseous nerve*
48. *Superficial branch of radial nerve – C5, C6, C7, C8*
49. *Ulnar nerve – C7, C8, T1*
50. *Median nerve – C5, C6, C7, C8, T1*
51. *Dorsal digital nerve*
52. *Median nerve*

It was a very significant time for Lizzie who excitedly told me that the British Medical Journal had just published the results of a 12 month trial in which Alexander Technique had been tested against usual treatments for back pain and had scored so favourably that she felt there was a strong possibility that funding would be more forthcoming in the future and that Alexander Technique may be more accessible on the NHS.

📖 **For press article on Alexander Technique see page 200**

The trial refers to back pain, but of course since our backs support us and our nervous systems, they are pivotal to general health. It was only when I started to research this book and I came across anatomical drawings like the one on page 140, which show the nervous system that I realised how big some of the nerves are and I hadn't had any real idea previously of the way they are housed in the spinal column. I only had only a vague notion.

The image and component information on the previous two pages are taken from an anatomical chart which can be bought as a poster (with various mounting styles) or a laminated fold up study guide measuring 23 cm × 10.4 cm when folded.

📖 **For Anatomical Chart Company see page 239**

I found these drawings really fascinating, and they helped me enormously to understand the structure of the nervous system and particularly in relation to the Alexander Technique where there is great emphasis on the neck and spine. For me the Alexander Technique sessions worked perfectly with all the other treatments.

It was now summer and due to continual effort and exercise on the part of 'my team' we were finding that the accumulative effects were at last beginning to show. I was instinctively attempting to use my hand all-be-it restrictively to perform day to day tasks. This was a turning point because in spite of the swelling and pain it now felt as though it had life in it (approx 30% movement). It really highlighted for me how all the treatments had worked together against the crippling symptoms of the CRPS. I hope that I have given enough information to stimulate an interest in the therapies in the context of CRPS treatments.

Mr Lakhani and Osteopathy

Elizabeth has regular treatment for her arthritis with an Ayurvedic practitioner. She urged me to come with her to an appointment where she introduced me to Rebecca, the practitioner. When Rebecca saw my hand she studied it carefully and then wrote down the name of a Mr Lakhani whose practice is in North Finchley. He had apparently alleviated a chronic slipped disc in her mother in law's neck, she, having had no luck with other therapies for over two years. I have to say at this stage I felt reluctant to go to yet another practitioner, but a few weeks later after some bouts of very nasty muscle spasms, I made an appointment.

I arrived for my first appointment at a very unassuming practice in a house in North Finchley. I was not really sure what was about to happen, but had a lot of faith in Elizabeth's Ayurvedic practitioner whose work with her was so successful. It is very unlike me not to be more enquiring, but I think I imagined I was going for an Ayurvedic massage. When I saw the plaques on the wall, I realised that Mr Lakhani was an Osteopath. I was horrified as in the past before I found Alexander Technique I had had a rather traumatic experience with an Osteopath, who I later found out was not registered with any regulatory organisation and I had vowed that I would never allow anyone to crunch my bones ever again. When Mr Lakhani showed me into the therapy room, I immediately explained that I was in the wrong place and that I didn't need an Osteopath and I was willing to pay for the appointment, but would like to excuse myself and leave. He chuckled and asked me why I felt this way and I mumbled something about my hand being the problem and he assured me that it was all connected and asked me to sit down and we began to talk about all my symptoms, the accident with the pot and the treatments I had already received. He guided me through an intensive history of accidents, health issues, and emotional issues, all of which he explained could cause long term imbalances and trauma. I was still, at this point having to wear the odema glove most of the time to avoid my hand swelling. By the time Mr Lakhani began the treatment I felt very confident that he might be able to help me.

Instead of doing bone crunching, he worked on the soft tissue on my shoulder and arm and also on my ribs and spine. He did very little to my hand on that first appointment. The treatment lasted over an hour and he seemed in no rush but remained focussed on what he was doing. Afterwards I was still very tender but I was also conscious of a sense that something had changed for the better.

At the end of that first session Mr Lakhani gave me some hand exercises and advised me to rub arnica cream on my shoulder and back where he had been working. He also told me to use a hot water bottle on my shoulder and alternate it with something very cold from the freezer (perhaps frozen peas). I told him that I had problems with pain in the night as it was difficult to find an appropriate position for my shoulder. He took out a V Pillow which appears earlier in the book.

📖 **For more information on V Pillow see pages 37 and 239**

I knew immediately after the treatment that there had been a shift in what was happening in my arm and I made another appointment. The hand exercise was invaluable and produced a significant result in the movement of my wrist. This exercise had been impossible up until this point. It could be done passively but not actively.

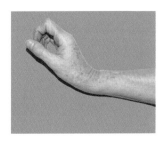
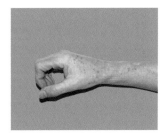
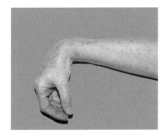

On my second appointment after some treatment to my shoulder, Mr Lakhani began working on my fingers. Although they were still very sensitive and at times painful, once I let go of my fear and considered my breathing and calmed myself down, I realised that I wouldn't have come back unless I trusted what he was doing. With that in mind I completely relaxed as he worked on me. After that appointment there was a notable change to my shoulder and I found myself able to spend time without the oedema glove which had become a full time accessory. Within that month I was able to shed it completely as the circulation in my hand was markedly improved and I was able to do more challenging exercises, both with Joseph and at home.

Psychologically it was a huge step for me to shed the oedema glove, because it acted like a signal of my condition, both to others and to myself. When I was dressing to go out, it would be my last act, donning the glove. It made me feel safe, that my still painful hand was protected, but it also drew attention from others and I was becoming tired of telling the story. Before my visits to Mr Lakhani when I left the glove off, my hand would swell and turn purple unless I kept it in 'the wave position'.

This was no longer the case, but I realised now that there was a slight resistance to taking it off because it had been a symbol of my pain and it had protected my hand so well over the last year. To take it off would leave my hand exposed and that was quite a frightening prospect. I very quickly got over that once the glove was off and thanks to Mr Lakhani's Osteopathy, the painful effects of the oedema subsided as my circulation improved and I celebrate every day all the things I can do. Nobody notices that there are restrictions on what I can do and that's helpful in complete recovery, because body language is so important in how we are viewed. The racking pain for all that time had often produced some pretty unusual body language.

I saw Mr Lakhani 8 times, during which the actual 'bone crunching' occupied, all in all, less than a minute. Now in the hands of a regulated Osteopath with experience, I was no longer afraid of the moment of manipulation and discarded the phrase 'bone crunching' which belonged in the past to my bad experience. Mr Lakhani is passionate about his work and like Joseph celebrated my progress. After the second treatment which had lasted an hour and a half, where he had worked on my hand, and freed up the fingers a little, the circulation certainly improved and so did the movement in my arm and shoulder. After another two sessions my shoulder was almost completely pain free. Mr Lakhani has given me cranial Osteopathy treatment and has treated my damaged knees and I am happy to say that since the circulation has improved and there is no longer an oedema problem I am able to really exercise my hand and fingers. I still have to do this as many times as possible during the day and if I wake up at night, but if this is as good as it gets, this is good enough for me. The extraordinarily positive results achieved through the work of Mr Lakhani made me rethink the necessity of returning to Taiwan and in the end I decided that further CMT treatment was no longer necessary. I will be eternally grateful to Dr. Ko and Dr. Wang. Everything that I have achieved since returning from Taiwan was only possible due to their alleviation of the most profound level of pain that I was experiencing prior to the CMT treatment. However, these holistic treatments can be used in different combinations at different times in the treatment regime. Each patient is unique. The important thing is to find the right practitioner.

I continued to see Joseph regularly at the Occupational Therapy unit and he in turn continued to show me that he was not in the slightest bit jealous of my work with other practitioners. In fact he was genuinely excited about the progress in my hand and was always interested to know what the other therapies had consisted of.

Now that I was able to use my hand for more and more activities I had noticed that if I wrote with my right hand I would be unaware of the amount of pressure that I was applying to the pen. There would be a deep groove in my finger from it when I had finished writing. Likewise if I held the phone in that hand when I was finished talking I would notice dark red pressure marks where I had gripped the receiver. I mentioned this to Joseph and as usual he understood what I was describing and told me that it was quite a common occurrence and brought out a small gauge attached to a rubber bulb.

The idea is that when you squeeze the bulb it records your grip strength. Joseph suggested that I did not try to test my grip strength, but instead squeeze it just enough to trigger the gauge and then try and maintain the grip to keep the same pressure. It was an excellent exercise and I discovered I had no control at all. Even if I really concentrated it was pretty impossible. He asked me to take the device home with me and work on it as often as I could. It certainly helped to make me conscious of over gripping, and it did improve over time from actively working on it with Joseph's gauge but even now, I still at times find myself applying too much pressure to a toothbrush or hairbrush or some other object.

Now when the pains came they were nothing like the intensity that they had been. They were strange and felt more like wind blowing over an ember, but not firing it, so although I braced myself for the onslaught of the pain, it would die out. When I described this to Joseph he explained to me in a simple way how to view what was happening. He told me that the extreme pain would have created, over the long period, substantial neural pathways. Now that there was significant healing and a lot more movement, most of that pain had diminished. However whatever pain there was would still travel up these enlarged pathways and so my body would brace itself in anticipation of the agony to the extent that even my face would grimace, ready for the blitz, but the message was much smaller than the pathway.

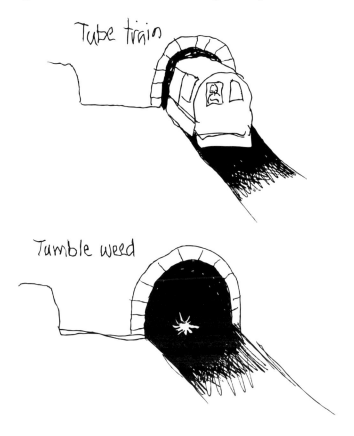

I was very excited by this information. It appealed to me visually and I imagined a tube train entering a station and how it fills up the tunnel and then I imagined a tumble weed being blown down the tunnel and bouncing off the sides but losing momentum. This became the way I viewed the lessening pain signals and made a conscious effort not to grimace when they began, but to breathe carefully and try to compose myself. I hoped this would help to narrow the neural pathways. It really worked for me psychologically and then physically.

Getting Back to Normal

As the second Christmas season since the accident approached I was able to really see the results of the treatments that I had been so fortunate to access. The pain in my hand had become completely manageable. Mr Lakhani's brilliant treatments which freed up my shoulder and allowed me to shed the oedema glove enabled great 'leaps' forward in the continued work with Joseph at the hand unit. The breakthroughs, which were now occurring weekly, and the general progress in movement was very exciting. Because of the nature of the crush injury there is virtually no movement in the knuckles of my middle and ring fingers. With a lot of work the tips of the index and little finger are more able to clutch.

In the New Year Joseph introduced me to the Biometrics method. In short this is a therapeutic tool which is interactive on a computer screen. They are like very simple computer games in which the patient, for instance, has to move a basket from side to side collecting balls which are dropping from the top of the screen. (For those who remember vintage computer games it is a bit like 'Space Invaders') The device to move the basket will either be a round wheel set like a small steering wheel sized appropriately for the stretch of one hand, fingers outstretched and gripping the edge of the wheel or a one resembling the accelerator on a motor bike and situated at the same angle as on a bike. This instrument provides a stretch and a movement for the wrist and fingers which I can't describe. The tightness of the 'accelerator' or 'steering wheel' can be adjusted depending on your level of treatment. I have to admit I am a bit competitive and the fact that the machine scores your 'game' is really rewarding, because you can set yourself targets and it will keep a record of your progress. There are so many exercises to do and by using your hand as much as possible you achieve some of the stretching, but these Biometric exercises worked miracles in awakening movement that had been dormant in my hand for the last year or so. It is so exciting when this kind of thing takes place.

It is important to note here that although the symptoms of the CRPS were no longer ripping through my hand, the process of relearning how to use it was in itself quite painful. I want to urge you not to lose hope and to keep up the movements and mirror work and exercises. It really pays off at times like this after so many months of the frustrating 'three steps forward and two steps back' routine when suddenly whole new movements are possible because of the accumulation of that work. Ask at your Occupational Therapy unit if they have a Biometric System. This was perfect timing for my hand at that time, but would have been impossible a few months before when I wouldn't have been able to stretch my hand enough to turn the wheel. It would have been much too painful.

It is very important to pace yourself and be aware of your limitations when doing exercises. If you achieve steady progress without over straining it is more likely that you might keep them up, whereas if you push yourself too hard and make the pain worse, you might be tempted to just give up altogether. This really applies to any exercise. I was to meet quite a few people when visiting Mr Lakhani who had injured themselves by not warming up correctly before doing really strenuous exercises in the gym. In the same way it is better to start slowly and work steadily when doing hand or foot exercises. This is why the wax bath is so good, because it helps a lot by warming and softening the joints before beginning therapy.

📖 **For more information on Wax Bath see pages 77 and 239**

Elizabeth continues to insist on the massages every time we are together. At this stage when she does it we can really notice the difference in movement and lack of general stiffness.

As I sit writing this my hand and arm feel absolutely normal. When I move and try to do things I am fully aware that there are still problems and very occasionally I still have the tugging feeling and for structural reasons my injured knuckles and fingers remain very stiff. Most of the time though, now that I no longer wear the oedema glove, I forget about it and just get on with my life. It is possible that I might go ahead and try to have a knuckle replacement. I would do this only because I still can't make a fist and so an important part of my hand is immobilised and therefore is laid open to arthritis and maybe eventual bone and muscle atrophy. It is still very stiff and at times the skin turns shiny and I feel a faint return of the gluey tugging feeling but none of the major harrowing symptoms remain. I touch wood.

I have been told that there is, unfortunately, a strong possibility that the CRPS could flare up again with the intervention of surgery. It's something I will have to decide upon over the next few months. When I last saw the Consultant she advised me to come for a follow up appointment around this time to review my situation and discuss possible surgery. Again I require a GP referral to this unit. As in my earlier encounters with my GP surgery *this* in itself is a 'painful' exercise.

After an extremely impersonal exchange I was told that I didn't need a referral since I had already been there on the 'CHOOSE and BOOK' method. I insisted that six months had passed and I was sure I needed a new referral. I was told to phone and make an appointment and if it didn't work to come back. I was so frustrated but agreed to drop in a letter if I did need the referral. Having called up the NHS hospital I was told that 6 months had lapsed and I did indeed need a new GP referral. So again I wrote to the GP explaining what had happened and again requesting a referral. A few days later I received a phone call from him asking me to remind him what the referral was for. I reminded him it was for my hand. As I write, that was three weeks ago and thankfully the referral has arrived in the post this morning. I include this little scenario, really to illustrate how without the support that I received, I may well have landed up with a very problematic hand and been a very long term drain on the health service. I think that the most upsetting aspect to this is that I realise that there are some out there who have CRPS or for that matter any painful disorder, who have to plough their way through a 'care system' which has largely removed time for care and replaced it with so much bureaucracy that often in my experience I have felt more like a prisoner before a parole board than a patient before a doctor.

I have to reiterate though that when I have found a department providing good care in the NHS it has been excellent – so it is possible.

Above all else try to get yourself into an Occupational Therapy Unit as soon as possible. They will help you to help yourself.

Generally though I am so thankful that the CRPS didn't move to any other location in my body and that I was able to endure the pain while working on the condition and that I didn't have to resort to a cocktail of pain medications. I am so grateful to Elizabeth and Shal, without whose passionate support, things for me could have been very different. I hope that this book has been useful and informative and I wish you well!

Please keep using and moving your limb. It is the single most important piece of advice I can give you. It is essential to healing even though just the idea of moving may terrify you in anicipation of the pain.

Think of the movement in your whole sytem.

In your mind's eye see your injury healed and your limb in use.

It has to be more positive than thinking of it as useless!

This was supposed to be the end of the book but…

DOUBLE WAVE POSITION

Having spent pretty well fifteen months dealing with the all encompassing effects of CRPS I felt so liberated having discarded the oedema glove and returned to 'normal pain free life'. I began working wholeheartedly on this book and went about my daily life as before.

About seven months later I was at a Film Festival and after dinner, as we walked back towards the car park through a public garden I tripped over a very low hooped fence, commonly found in parks. I went from the grass onto a concrete pathway and broke both my wrists. As my chin hit the ground I already knew that the wrists were broken.

Actually at first I felt extremely embarrassed because I figured that it would be difficult for anyone to take me seriously about the book now, with both hands in the wave position. I feared they might think me some sort of clown. I also felt really sorry for Elizabeth and Jeff and Don who were with me. The looks of shock on their faces as they tried to pick me up will be an enduring memory. Somehow being the patient is sometimes less traumatic than being a witness. All that quickly disappeared though as the reality of both hands out of action began playing itself out.

I am going to keep this brief because the message I want to deliver is that this new accident literally hurtled me into a fairly unique position. Having had a fracture and developed CRPS, then having managed to overcome it, I was now faced with two wrist fractures requiring surgery to install plates. I was told that approximately 20% of patients who undergo this surgery develop varying degrees of CRPS. The strange thing is that I didn't feel scared. I really had confidence that even if I did get it, all the things that I had learned on the first round would prevent me becoming a chronic case. There were however some extremely sobering moments and again I had the loving support of my friends who literally became my hands, another humbling experience for me as someone who up until recently always saw myself as strong and independent.

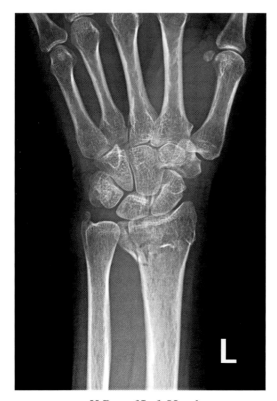
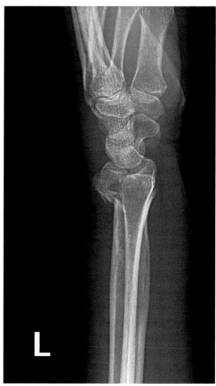

X Ray of Left Hand   *X Ray of Left Hand Profile*

The first couple of days after the accident I was very uncomfortable and the back slabs (plaster casts with bandage) were heavy.

As I mentioned above my girlfriends created a sort of rota to take turns in looking after me, so at this stage Mimi, who had driven down to Elizabeth's to fetch me had delivered me into the hands of Shal and Rob where I would stay for the next ten days or so.

The back slabs remained on until Shal and I went to see the consultant (three days later) who explained that surgery would be advisable for these kinds of breaks. My deciding question was whether or not movement would be hindered without surgery, since I already had residual difficulties which inhibited partial movement with my right hand resulting from the CRPS and the inevitable consequence of the crush injury.

📖 **For images on finger restrictions see page 120**

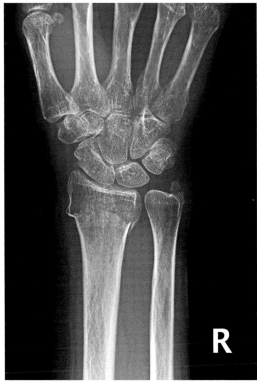

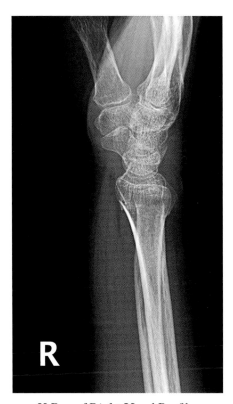

X Ray of Right Hand   *X Ray of Right Hand Profile*

I was told that successful surgery would help to rectify some of the restrictions of movement associated with these new breaks. I was again told that 20% of

patients undergoing wrist surgery developed some degree of CRPS. Since I had
already had CRPS there was some concern that it might return.

Coincidently I already had a hospital appointment with a view to discussing
the possible surgery to my right hand, so I was able to now take up that
appointment for the surgery to both. This luckily gave me two weeks to go
away and think about it and make a final decision.

I was duly fitted out with fibreglass casts on both hands. My right hand was
absolutely fine, but my left hand felt extremely tender and pretty much as
soon as I was in the cast, I began to experience some of the shooting pains
familiar to me from the CRPS. Before continuing with the casts another x ray
was done to see if there was any unnoticed injury to my knuckles, but there
were no such injuries. It was very strange sensation because the pains origi-
nated in exactly the same place as the crush injury nerve pains had been on my
other hand. Starting in the tips of my middle, ring and little fingers, they shot
up my hand into my wrist and into my elbow. By the evening the left hand
was very swollen and I could feel the pressure of the cast. Shal gave me some
Ibuprofen and Paracetamol which helped a little, but by morning my hand was
like a blown up rubber glove emerging from the cast and was a familiar bluish
colour. It was quite a strange experience because Joseph had talked to me about
neural pathways. Now I seemed to be experiencing a sort of mirror reaction
and identical neural pathways appeared to be operating in my left hand that
had been involved in the pain on my right hand during the CRPS. Mystifying
really since the fractures this time were to the big bones at my wrists.

I think the gods must have been with me at this stage, because like my coinci-
dental appointment for surgery, I also had an outstanding appointment to see
Mr Lakhani the day after having the casts fitted. This was really supposed to
have been a final six monthly follow up appointment since the removal of the
oedema glove and my return to normal life. The appointment had been made
six weeks earlier.

So between feeling rather resigned to the return of the pain and vaguely hopeful that Mr Lakhani would be able to at least advise me on what to do, a friend
drove me to the appointment. I didn't imagine for one minute that he would be
able to intervene and reduce the swelling and stop the pain at that stage. I felt
quite afraid as I lay on the treatment bed, even though I trust Mr Lakhani implicitly. After an hour and a half of cranial work and tissue massage my friend

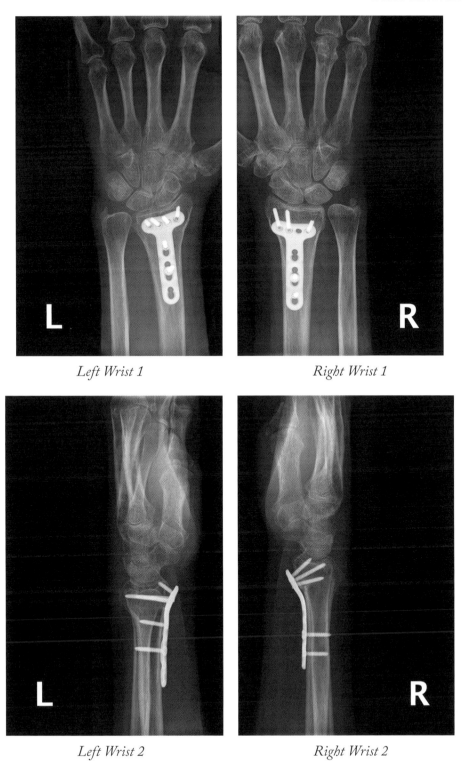

Left Wrist 1   *Right Wrist 1*

Left Wrist 2   *Right Wrist 2*

drove me back to Shal's. I always feel much 'lighter' after Mr Lakhani's treatments, but I couldn't have expected that by the time we got back the swelling would have completely gone. Shal opened the door to us when we got back and excitedly pointed out that my hand had shrunk and was no longer puffing over the plaster. The normal colour had returned and by later that afternoon there was no longer any pressure from the cast, or any shooting pains or any other pains for that matter. Neither the extreme swelling nor the pains have returned at any point.

I had by now decided to go ahead with surgery. I made my decision based on the distortions I had felt in both wrists on the night of my accident and the prognosis of the Consultant that without surgery there would be hindrance to some movement. Since my right hand already had various restrictions, I was keen to try to achieve as much movement as possible after this new accident. I felt that since my bone density is good, I would put myself in the hands of the Consultant and her team because I trusted her. She had explained that they would insert a plate on to the radius in both wrists. These plates would help to re-align the head of radius which would ultimately, with extensive Hand Therapy and exercise, restore wrist movement.

So in just over three weeks from the date of 'the fall' I was in surgery. The NHS Hospital was modern and clean and everyone in the Treatment Centre was professional and empathic. It was a completely uplifting environment. Whereas I had felt a bit apprehensive about the surgery, I now felt quite calm. People within the surgical team commented on the fact that there was an unusual absence of swelling.

As the anaesthetist installed the port she mentioned that she had heard me talking to the Consultant about this book. She asked what it was about and I said "CRPS but unless you know what that is it is a long story."

"I have time." She said. I began "Well CRPS sssssssss *zzzzzzzzzzzzzzzzzz*"

When I woke up after surgery I had the usual nausea and unsteadiness associated with general anaesthetic. Both arms were elevated and strapped to stands on either side of the bed. I felt like one of those classic joke characters in traction. I drifted in and out of sleep for most of the day. Shal was at my bedside all day to help me to drink. I immediately began trying gently to straighten my fingers and have kept up exercising ever since.

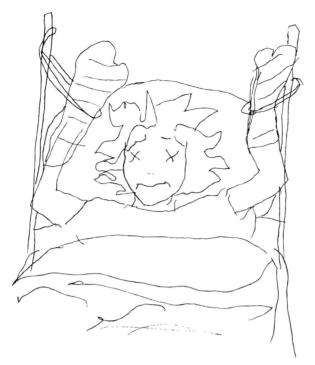

I felt like some sort of joke character

Without going into too many unnecessary details, my night in the ward was horrendous to the point that if I could have got out of there I would have. I had the feeling that the nurses were probably agency people who went from hospital to hospital and so no routine appeared to be in place. I felt incredibly helpless and vulnerable and had an inkling of what it must be like to be in long term care when you are unable to do anything for yourself and how demeaning that can be.

If you are unhappy with your treatment find out the complaints route and write or email them giving as many details as possible.

This appears to work because what follows is an account of my complaint and the results: I left the hospital the day after surgery and as soon as I was able I wrote an email to PAL – The Patient Advice and Liaison Office – outlining every detail of my horrendous night on the ward. I was contacted within an hour thanking me and informing me that a copy of my email had been forwarded to the Ward Sister and to all the other departments who I had actually mentioned very favourably – The Treatment Centre, where I had had surgery, The Outpatients Clinic, The Hand Therapy Outpatients and The Radiology Department all of who were fantastically well run and had excellent customer care.

When I had left the ward in question, I had been asked to rate my care at the hospital. This was to be done on a sort of electronic device with multiple choice answers – e.g: a) excellent – b) good – c) satisfactory etc. Firstly I didn't have the use of either of my hands, so my friend who had come to collect me punched in the answers. Secondly there was no differentiation between the Surgery Unit, the Radiology Unit or any other for that matter. It was a sort of overall comment on the hospital which had little value in really assessing where there may have been problems. I put all of these points in the email. Very shortly after that I received an email from the Ward sister inviting me to a meeting which would be held to discuss the findings of an investigation into my complaint. I went to the meeting and found it very useful. Each section of my complaint had been highlighted and we discussed them in detail. They thanked me for making such a detailed complaint, because it gave them clear objectives to pursue. They explained what was to be done to rectify some of the issues I had outlined and explained other issues which were to do with hospital procedure and which were in place for the safety benefit of the patients. I felt really pleased that I had gone and I received a follow up letter outlining the various suggestions which had arisen out of the meeting and how they were going to be addressed on the ward.

The tip is that if you can follow up on your complaint, it is possible that it could make a difference.

📖 **For more information on The Patient Advice and Liaison Office see page 169**

Meanwhile I was fast learning how it is to be completely dependent on others for **everything**! I will let you use your imagination.

This time I decided to take some of the strong pain killers and sleep as much as possible until I could go back to the hospital and have splints installed. I wanted to try and recover as quickly as possible and get on with this book. I did however try to move my fingers as much as was possible within the very heavy 'back slabs'.

Ok let's be clear on this! So, strong painkillers = constipation, particularly if you are not moving around very much.

Prepare yourself for this horrible eventuality. Ask who ever prescribes the pain-killers to give you something for the constipation, ask about Milk of Magnesia, prune juice, dried apricots, dried prunes or senna pods. Don't allow it to get chronic; it is sooo painful and really bad for your recovery. It is your plumbing! Make sure you drink *plenty* of water. Constipation can cause problems which untreated have long term consequences, like anal fissures (a small tear in the skin around the anus). These tears are the result of straining. I have spoken to so many people who have had this as a result of constipation after a course of strong painkillers. **Discuss this with your GP or whoever is treating you.**

So meanwhile I was now in the double wave position and feeling really silly. After the splints were on they actually looked a bit like a fashion accessory, because people can't really imagine that you could break both hands! My friends were fantastically supportive as usual and patiently helped me to bath, dress, eat – pretty much everything as I said above.

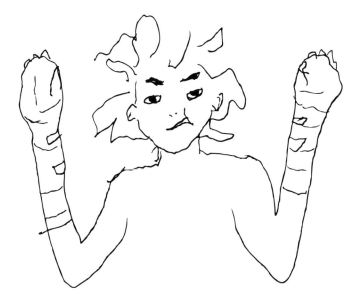

Five days after surgery the back slabs were removed and splints were made for me at the Physiotherapy Hand Unit at the hospital. I was treated there by a very conscientious Physiotherapist who was another person I was grateful to have had treating me. She was very patient and a couple of times when I had had to return in between appointments because of pressure points on the splints, she had even stayed late to see me and made sure that those points were loosened and padded.

I have discovered by talking to others who have CRPS that many believe it was the rubbing of an ill fitting cast on pressure points that not only caused them the most excruciating pain but contributed to the CRPS.

This time round, the Hand Therapy in general was very different, because after surgery I was not allowed to do anything which involved resistance. Which meant NO opening of doors, slicing food, pulling on socks or shoes, brushing teeth – or just about everything you can think of. The second big no was to lifting anything, which even included half a cup of tea – absolutely NO LIFTING. Very frustrating! For the first few weeks I was completely dependent on friends. There were lots of active movements allowed. The Physiotherapist gave me many exercises to do, which I really worked on since there was very little else that I could do.

straighten hand   *hook position*   *bend knuckles*   *make a fist*

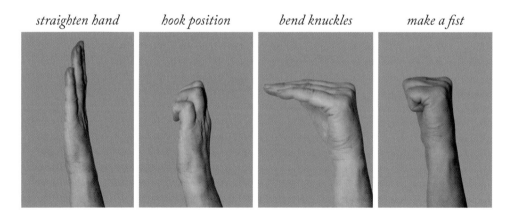

After a few weeks she gave me a particularly useful exercise using playing cards which helped my wrists to rotate. As always it was very slow at first, but got easier with practice. I continue this exercise even now, months after the accident.

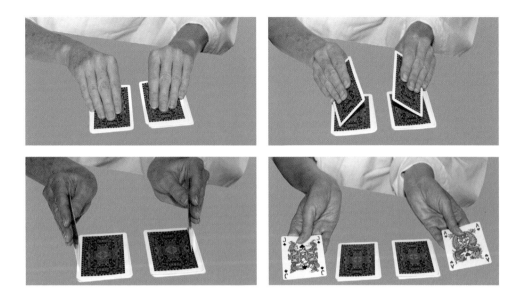

She also emphasised how important it is to massage, or in my case ask someone to massage the surgery scars to soften them. Obviously this is something which your Hand Therapist will suggest when it is the appropriate time. The therapist treating me suggested I use a non-perfumed cream (vitamin E cream is good) and pressing down quite deep and hard on the scar, make small circular movements across and around the scar and continue to do this often during the day. Ideally accumulatively these little massage sessions (roughly 5–10 minutes) should make up at least an hour a day. At first I found it a bit scary, touching and pushing down on a recent wound, but she explained it was very important that the scarring did not attach to the underlying tissues and structures in the wrist. So the idea was to stretch and keep the scar tissue moving. Scars are produced as the body is involved in normal healing process. They consist of blood vessels, cells and fibrous tissue. Scars can hinder movement in the long term and can pucker the skin around them. I was very grateful that I knew about this because I noticed that the scar appeared to be quite minimal post operatively, and then changed and became thicker, redder and more raised. Again friends massaged my scars conscientiously and it really paid off.

I thought so much about amputees and in particular soldiers who are coming back from the two current wars with horrendous bomb blast injuries. One minute they are on the battlefield and the next they are totally dependent on others for their every move. I know how it affected me psychologically, but my injuries were miniscule in comparison. Again I was aware of the incredible job Occupational Therapists and Physiotherapists do. It should never be underestimated.

The two V Pillows, which I was now using, were absolute life savers as far as sleeping comfortably was concerned. Friends who were taking care of me each acquired a pair for me to use when I stayed over in their care.
As I have mentioned before the pillows are so light and easy to lift because of their shape. I cannot recommend them too highly.

Meanwhile, I tried as soon as possible to venture out on my own. At first it was very scary because with the knowledge that I didn't have the use of my hands, it felt a bit unbalanced and there was a tendency to be over cautious which in itself put me off balance even further.
It took quite a few weeks to get over the fear of falling again. There were added complications in that when I travelled on the underground I had to be careful not to try and get up until the train had stopped because I couldn't hold on. Going up and down escalators felt precarious with the knowledge that I had no way of gripping. Buses were a complete no-no. Often the drivers seem to relish throwing their passengers around and if you are not in your seat quickly enough you are in trouble and could easily fall over. This I had discovered during my bout of CRPS. Using only one hand I had often been thrown against a vertical hand rail or another passenger and suffered the intensely painful circumstances. I had no intention of even attempting this method of transport during the first few months and so found myself walking more and more.

In due course I was referred back to Joseph because we already had a programme to continue working on the knuckles of my right hand after the CRPS. As usual, being treated in that Hand Unit was a pleasure and as usual Joseph showed me exercises to do which really helped to get movement into my wrists. Here is one which I particularly liked because you have to go down onto your haunches to do it. So you stand up and flatten your hand as much as possible on a table. Bring your arm horizontal, which will mean bending your knees and then go as far down as you can to give your wrist the full stretch. It is a very effective exercise and anyone trying it will feel the benefits.

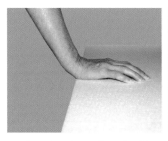 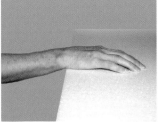 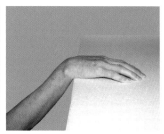

Rest hand on edge of table *Position arm horizontally* *Drop arm as low as possible*

I'd like to share another exercise which I found excellent to combat stiffness. Most people will have had some experience with a therapy ball or with the therapy sponge. It is a squeezing motion and at times, for me, is still uncomfortable, but it really works to strengthen the fingers and gives a good stretch. I recommend it. Your Hand Therapist will give you the correct colour sponge for appropriate density. In the beginning even the least dense one was agony and I couldn't squeeze it at all, now I use all three.

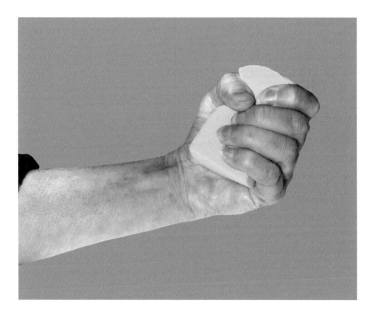

Above all try to do everything you normally would with your hands. Even if at first it seems that you are too weak to complete the task, persevere the next day and so on, it is so rewarding. Whereas the devices shown earlier will help with immediate difficulties or long term illnesses which make certain movements impossible, trying to get back to normal activity is so psychologically important and gratifying. Opening a can, managing to peel an apple, or pulling a plug out of a socket can be cause for extreme celebration. Please try it!

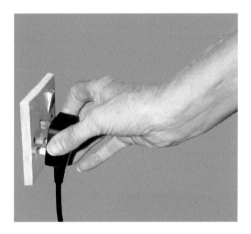

Recovery for me was quite swift this time round thanks to the combination of Occupational Therapy and Mr Lakhani's Cranial Osteopathy and I am pleased to say that my wrists are recovering well and so the book is finished. I know that I will have to keep up the exercises that I have been given for a very long time. I still feel the stiffness every morning when I wake up, but at least I know that I can work at it and hopefully prevent any long term nasty conditions which arise out of the immobility in my knuckle joints.

Mirror therapy was no longer an option since both hands were injured. It is important to note again that visual feedback using mirrors requires a healthy limb to reflect.

I hope that the telling of my experiences will be useful to anyone involved in any way with CRPS/RSD or any kind of pain, whether the Patient or the Health Professional.

The End

Tips and Health Information

If you don't have computer access, Public Libraries have computers and the librarians will assist you to use them. This is handy if you want to look up anything to do with your health.

Register with the Patients Association (see page 209) to receive newsletters and find out all the campaigns they are running on behalf of patients. They really are brilliant.

You can ask at your GP surgery or Public Library for the phone numbers or addresses of your local NHS, so you could phone or write, requesting information. Don't be afraid to ask, it is your choice! The NHS has a great website (**www.nhs.uk**) that you can visit which will help you get many answers to your questions. The following important information is from their site.

○○○○○

Accessing your health Records
Under the Data Protection Act 1998, you have a legal right to access your health records. If you want to see your health records you can ask at your GP surgery and arrange a time to come in and read them. You don't have to give a reason for wanting to see your records.

If you want to see your health records you may be asked to submit your request in writing. It's a good idea to state the dates of the records that you want to see – for example, from 2000 to 3000 – and then send the letter by recorded delivery. You should also keep a copy of your letter for your records. You will usually receive a response to your request within 21 days, although the law states that your hospital or surgery has up to 40 days to respond.

Hospital records

As well as having a copy of your health records, your GP surgery will also have a summary of any hospital tests or treatment that you have had. Any hospitals where you have had treatment or tests will also hold records. To see your hospital health records, you will have to contact your local Hospital Trust. Your request to see your records will be forwarded to the health records manager. The manager will decide whether your request will be approved. Your request will usually only be refused if your records manager, GP, or other health professional believes the information in the records is likely to cause you, or another person, serious harm.

Charges

If your records have been updated in the last 40 days – that is, you have seen your GP or another health professional in the last 40 days, you're entitled to see your records free of charge. However, if your records are held on a computer, there may be an administration charge of up to £10.

For a copy of older paper records and results such as X-rays, you may have to pay photocopying and administration charges. These charges will be a maximum of £50 (in total) You should ask your surgery or hospital what they charge before you make a request.

Optician and dental records

Your optician and dental also hold records about you. To access your optician or dental records, you may need to show proof of identity.

Power of Attorney

Your health records are confidential and members of your family are not allowed to see them, unless you give them written permission, or they have power of attorney.

source: **www.nhs.uk**

Crown copyright material reproduced with permission of the controller HMSO

The Patient Advice and Liaison Service – pals

The NHS employs over a million staff in thousands of locations. It is a large and complex organisation providing a broad range of services. It is not surprising that sometimes you or a loved one may feel bewildered or concerned when using the NHS. And this can be at times when you are feeling at your most vulnerable and anxious.

So, what should you do if you want on the spot help when using the health service? The NHS expects all members of staff to listen and respond to you to the best of their ability. But sometimes, you may wish to talk to someone employed especially to help you. The Patient Advice and Liaison Service, known as PALS, has been introduced to ensure that the NHS listens to patients, their relatives, carers and friends, and answers their questions and resolves their concerns as quickly as possible.

PALS also helps the NHS to improve services by listening to what matters to patients and their loved ones and making changes, when appropriate.

What does PALS do?
In particular, PALS will:
- Provide you with information about the NHS and help you with any other health-related enquiry
- Help resolve concerns or problems when you are using the NHS
- Provide information about the NHS complaints procedure and how to get independent help if you decide you may want to make a complaint
- Provide you with information and help introduce you to agencies and support groups outside the NHS
- Inform you about how you can get more involved in your own healthcare and the NHS locally
- Improve the NHS by listening to your concerns, suggestions and experiences and ensuring that people who design and manage services are aware of the issues you raise
- Provide an early warning system for NHS Trusts and monitoring bodies by identifying problems or gaps in services and reporting them.

© PALS, author: Mr. Graeme A Calder, **www.pals.nhs.uk**
Ask your GP for local PALS Office Information or visit the website.

I found the following information on a leaflet in a local chemist. It is produced for the NHS and it gives constructive advice to patients.

Questions to ask
Before leaving your appointment, make sure you know the following:

What might be wrong? You could ask the following questions:
- Can I check that I have understood what you said? What you're saying is…
- Can you explain it again? I still don't understand.
- Can I have a copy of any letters written about me?

What about any further tests, such as blood tests, scans and so on?
- What are the tests for?
- How and when will I get the results?
- Who do I contact if I don't get the results?

About what treatment, if any, is best for you
- Are there other ways to treat my condition?
- What do you recommend?
- Are there any side effects or risks?
- How long will I need treatment for?
- How will I know if the treatment is working?
- How effective is this treatment?
- What will happen if I don't have any treatment?
- Is there anything I should stop or avoid doing?
- Is there anything else I can do to help myself?

What happens next and who to contact
- What happens next? Do I come back and see you?
- Who do I contact if things get worse?
- Do you have any written information?
- Where can I go for more information, a support group or more help?

Top tips
Before your appointment
- Write down your two or three most important questions.

- List or bring all your medicines and pills – including vitamins and supplements.
- Write down details of your symptoms, including when they started and what makes them better or worse.
- Ask your hospital or surgery for an interpreter or communication support if needed.
- Ask a friend or family member to come with you, if you like.

During your appointment
- Don't be afraid to ask if you don't understand. For example, "Can you say that again? I still don't understand."
- If you don't understand any words, ask for them to be written down and explained.
- Write things down, or ask a family member or friend to take notes.

Before you leave your appointment
Check that:
- ✓ you've covered everything on your list.
- ✓ you understand, for example "Can I just check I understood what you said?"
- ✓ you know what should happen next – and when. Write it down.

Ask:
- ✓ who to contact if you have any more problems or questions
- ✓ about support groups and where to go for reliable information, and
- ✓ for copies of letters written about you – you are entitled to see these.

After your appointment, don't forget the following:
- Write down what you discussed and what happens next. Keep your notes.
- Book any tests that you can and put the dates in your diary.

Ask:
- ✓ "what's happening if I am not sent my appointment details?" and
- ✓ "can I have the results of any tests?" (If you don't get the results when you expect – ask for them) Ask what the results mean.

Crown copyright material reproduced with permission of the controller HMSO

Mirror Visual Feedback Trial

A controlled pilot study of the utility of mirror visual feedback in the treatment of Complex Regional Pain Syndrome (type I)

**C. S. McCabe, R. C. Haigh, E. F. J. Ring, P. W. Halligan,[1]
P. D. Wall[2] and D. R. Blake**
The Royal National Hospital for Rheumatic Diseases in conjunction with The Department of Medical Sciences and The Department of Pharmacy and Pharmacology, University of Bath, Bath BAI IRL,
1 School of Psychology, University of Cardiff, PO Box 901, Cardiff CF10 3YG
2 Centre for Neuroscience Research, Hodgkin Building, King's College, London SEI IUL, UK

Abstract

Background. We assessed mirror visual feedback (MVF) to test the hypothesis that incongruence between motor output and sensory input produces complex regional pain syndrome (CRPS) (type I) pain.

Methods. Eight subjects (disease duration ≥3 weeks to ≤3 yr) were studied over 6 weeks with assessments including two controls (no device and viewing a non-reflective surface) and the intervention (MVF). Pain severity and vasomotor changes were recorded.

Results. The control stages had no analgesic effect. MVF in early CRPS (≤8 weeks) had an immediate analgesic effect and in intermediate disease (≤1 yr) led to a reduction in stiffness. At 6 weeks, normalization of function and thermal differences had occurred (early and intermediate disease). No change was found in chronic CRPS.

Conclusions. In early CRPS (type 1), visual input from a moving, unaffected limb re-establishes the pain-free relationship between sensory feedback and motor execution. Trophic changes and a less plastic neural pathway preclude this in chronic disease.

Key words: Complex regional pain syndrome, Mirror visual feedback.

Introduction

Complex regional pain syndrome (CRPS) is a painful, debilitating condition. This diagnostic term embraces several syndromes, including reflex sympathetic dystrophy, causalgia and algodystrophy. Characteristic clinical features include sensory disturbances, such as burning pain with allodynia and hyperalgesia; motor disturbances, such as weakness, tremor and muscle spasms; and changes in vascular tone, temperature and oedema [1]. Over time, functional loss and trophic changes may occur. The syndrome can occur spontaneously or following trauma (CRPS type 1) or in association with peripheral nerve damage (CRPS type 2). This paper addresses patients presenting with CRPS type 1.

A characteristic feature of CRPS is that signs and symptoms spread beyond the site of initial insult. Severe pain may occur seemingly out of proportion to the original pathology. It may persist over long periods and is frequently resistant to a wide range of treatments. Traditionally, interrupting the sympathetic supply to the painful area was thought to treat such pain. However, the effectiveness of this approach is not supported by randomized controlled trials [2]. Recent studies on other intractable pain conditions have reported the analgesic benefits of mirror visual feedback therapy [3]. Phantom limb pain, relieved by this therapy, has many characteristics similar to CRPS pain (burning, cramping, and mislocalized). We therefore investigated the effect of mirror visual feedback in CRPS.

The classical picture of a pain mechanism as a single hard-wired, dedicated pathway is no longer widely held [4, 5]. Instead, converging evidence from physiological and functional imaging studies suggests a much more diffuse and plastic system involving the cord, brainstem, thalamus and cortex [6]. In addition, psychological states such as attention, anticipation and preparation for action may be inherent, essential components modulating the experience of pain. Abnormal plastic changes in the central nervous system (CNS) have been associated with a number of pain syndromes [7, 8] including phantom limb pain [9]. For example, using non-invasive neuromagnetic imaging, Flor *et al*. [10] found a strong relationship between the amount of plastic change in primary somatosensory cortex and the extent of phantom pain experienced.

Ramachandran and Roger-Ramachandran [3] proposed that phantom limb pain results from disruption of the normal interaction between motor intention to move the limb and the absence of appropriate sensory (proprioceptive) feedback. They speculated that visual feedback might interrupt this pathological cycle. Using a mirror that enabled amputees to superimpose the visual image of their normal limb on the location where they felt their phantom limb to exist, Ramachandran and Roger-Ramachandran [3] found that the phantom spasms and their associated pain were rapidly relieved during exercises involving the 'virtual limb' in six out of 12 cases. Harris subsequently hypothesized, on the basis of clinical observation and functional imaging studies [11], that disorganized cortical representations may lead to the experience of peripheral pain. He proposed that a mismatch between motor intention and predicted proprioceptive or visual feedback of the affected limb may drive this process [12].

We hypothesized that the pain of CRPS is a consequence of disruption of central sensory processing and that congruent visual feedback from the moving unaffected limb, as provided by a mirror, would restore the integrity of cortical processing, thereby relieving pain and restoring function in the affected limb.

Method
Participants
Adult subjects who conformed to the diagnostic criteria for CRPS type 1 [1] in a single limb were recruited consecutively from the out-patient clinics at the Royal National Hospital for Rheumatic Diseases, Bath over an 18-month period. We excluded patients with CRPS type 2, for example those with peripheral nerve lesions.

Clinical method

Subjects were assessed at two time points: on presentation and 6 weeks later. The assessment protocol was divided into three distinct stages: two control phases (using no device and viewing a non-reflective surface) and an intervention phase (viewing a mirror). An additional daily diary was used to record frequency of mirror use and pain severity between assessments. Visual analogue scales (VAS) were used to assess pain intensity, with 0 = no pain and 10 = pain as bad as it could be. Infrared thermography (IRT) was used to quantify vasomotor changes that influenced temperature in the affected and unaffected limbs [13]. Images were taken on presentation and at week 6.

Subjects were seated and initially asked to visualize both limbs (affected and unaffected). Pain at rest and on movement was recorded (control phase 1). A non-reflective board was then positioned perpendicular to the subject's midline, with the unaffected limb facing the non-reflective surface and the affected limb hidden (control phase 2). Subjects were asked to attend to the non-reflective surface for a period of 5 min and exercise their non-painful limb and, if possible, their painful limb in a congruent manner (Fig. 1).

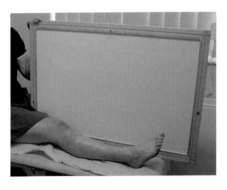 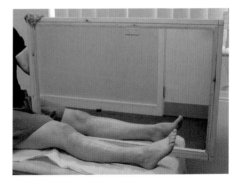

Fig. 1: Subject viewing non-reflective surface with painful limb hidden.   *Fig. 2: Subject viewing non-painful limb in mirror with painful limb hidden.*

All subjects were asked to attempt to perform similar exercises: flexion-extension cycles of the relevant body parts. The range of movement and speed of these exercises was dictated by the subject's pain. Following the control stages, a mirror of similar size to the control device was positioned so that only the unaffected limb, and its reflected image in the mirror, could now be seen (Fig. 2). Subjects attended to the reflection now occupying the space of their painful limb. Again, subjects were requested to exercise both limbs (flexion-extension cycles as described above) for 5 min in a congruent manner. Pain on movement was recorded after each control and intervention stage.

Following the initial procedures, subjects were directed to use the mirror as frequently as they wished. A maximum time limit of 10 min was set for each period of mirror therapy to ensure concentration was maintained. Subjects were also advised to conduct the treatment protocol in a quiet environment, where concentration would not be interrupted. Subjects recorded daily the frequency of mirror use and their movement-related pain score.

Results
(Table 1) Eight subjects were recruited, aged 24–40 yr (mean 33 yr) with disease duration of 3 weeks to 3 yr. Three subjects had early disease (≤8 weeks), two had disease of intermediate duration (5 months and 1 yr) and the remaining three had long-standing disease (≥2 yr). CRPS was precipitated by trauma in four of the eight subjects (cases 3, 5, 7 and 8); no obvious precipitant was identified in the remaining four. Case 6 had a concurrent diagnosis of ankylosing spondylitis but there was no clinical or imaging evidence of synovitis or enthesopathy in the painful region. Case 7 had extensive ulcers on the affected limb and all three chronic cases (cases 6–8) had contracture deformities in the CRPS-affected limb due to prolonged immobility.

All presented with a single limb affected by allodynia, hyperalgesia, reduced movement with related pain and stiffness and vasomotor disturbances. The only exception to this was case 4, who reported severe stiffness of the limb with little pain on movement but met all other criteria.

All subjects had had previous interventions that did not relieve pain, including analgesia, physiotherapy modalities, sympathetic blocks, immobilization, transcutaneous electrical nerve stimulation, Osteopathy and Acupuncture (Table 2). The more chronic cases had received the greater number of interventions, which included sympathetic blocks and immobilization. Standard physiotherapy treatment was continued throughout the study period (Table 3) for all subjects except case 5, who had discontinued treatment prior to the start of the study due to lack of benefit. The analgesic type, dose and frequency remained constant during the pre-study period and throughout the study period for those with chronic disease (cases 6–8). However, cases 1–5 reduced their analgesic requirements as the study progressed and at the 6-week follow up only case 5 still required any form of analgesia, and this only intermittently.

Control stages

All subjects reported no relief of pain on movement when both limbs were visualized without a device or when the non-reflective surface was viewed. Indeed, movement exacerbated pain. Control phase 2 of the protocol (using a whiteboard in place of the mirror) was only performed at the initial assessment. The reason for this was that the participants who experienced an immediate analgesic response with the mirror were aware that the whiteboard trials were purely for control purposes. It therefore no longer worked as a fair control, and as the mirror was so clearly beneficial to these participants they were reluctant to continue with the whiteboard. In order to keep the protocol uniform across the study participants, this phase was dropped for the 6-week intervention stage.

Intervention stage

All three subjects with early CRPS (≤8 weeks) reported a striking reduction in their pain VAS during and after visual feedback of their moving, unaffected limb as provided by the mirror. A marked analgesic effect was observed within a few minutes of mirror use, followed by an abrupt return of pain when the mirror was removed initially. With repeated use (four to nine times daily, week 1), the period of analgesia extended progressively from a few minutes to hours, requiring less mirror use over the 6-week study period. At 6 weeks there was a reversal of vasomotor changes as measured by IRT, a return to normal function and no pain at rest or on movement. All three subjects felt they no longer required analgesic relief from the mirror and had stopped prior to assessment at 6 weeks (case 3, week 4; cases 1 and 2, week 6).

The two subjects with intermediate disease duration (5 months and 1 year; cases 4 and 5) reported that the mirror immediately eased their movement-related stiffness but there was no analgesic effect in case 5. They both reported that this reduction in stiffness facilitated movement and the effect lasted for increasing periods after use of the mirror. Although no objective data were collected on function, both subjects felt that by 6 weeks function had improved to such an extent that they were able to return to their usual manual occupations. Interestingly, despite the lack of analgesic effect during the mirror visual feedback procedure, case 5 reported reduced pain at the 6-week follow-up (VAS $\frac{6}{10}$ at presentation and $\frac{1}{10}$ at 6 weeks). Reversal of IRT temperature differences was recorded in case 4 at 6 weeks, and case 5 remained with no significant difference between the two affected limbs.

No subjective relief of pain and stiffness or reversal of IRT temperature differences was observed in the three subjects with chronic disease (≥ 2 yr) and they had all discontinued mirror use by the end of week 3 due to lack of effect.

Comment

Our observations, the first of their kind in CRPS, suggest that congruent visual feedback of the moving unaffected limb, via a mirror, significantly reduces the perception of pain in early CRPS (type 1) and stiffness in the intermediate stages of the disease. The extent of the analgesic effect surprised both patients and investigators. The abrupt return of pain and stiffness when the mirror was removed supports the view that we were reliably able to influence these sensations. The two internal control stages excluded an analgesic effect from (i) moving the affected limb with normal visual feedback alone and (ii) the influence of selective attention when the limb was hidden. A placebo response is therefore highly unlikely, given the above control stages and the lack of benefit in chronic CRPS subjects. The effect was consistent between the five less chronic subjects and repeatable within subjects. Extended use of the mirror provided increasing periods of analgesia, which aided compliance with exercise regimens. Whilst early CRPS can resolve spontaneously, we are unaware of any therapeutic manoeuvres or drug effects that can achieve such an immediate analgesic effect. In addition, when the intervention is stopped there is an abrupt return of pain. Mirror visual feedback is a simple, inexpensive and, most importantly, a patient-directed treatment.

Our results support the hypothesis that the CNS is capable of generating a feedback-dependent state that can produce pathological levels of pain. In CRPS, this might involve a mismatch between different interdependent modalities, such as a disruption of normal interaction between motor intention and sensory feedback. In those with inherent vulnerability to this incongruence it can lead, in some, to referred, intractable pain following trauma, and in others it can promote CRPS with a CNS origin. This might explain why some types of CRPS occur without discrete peripheral injury.

Subject, painful limb, age (yr), sex	Symptom duration	At presentation Mean temp difference: painful – non-painful limb (°C)[a]	Control phase 1[b] Pain VAS at rest	Control phase 1[b] Pain VAS on movement	Control phase 2[c] Pain VAS on movement	Intervention[d] Pain VAS on movement	Frequency of mirror use (times per day) (duration of each treatment 10 min) Week 1	Week 2	Week 3	Week 4	Week 5	Week 6	Follow-up At 6 weeks Pain VAS	Mean temp. diff. (°C)	Treatment duration (weeks)
1, LL, 38, F	6 weeks	1.1	9	9	9	2	8	3	3	3	2	0	0	0.2	6
2, LA, 28, F	3 weeks	2.0	7	8	8	3	4	4	3	3	2	0	0	0.4	6
3, LL, 34, F	8 weeks	2.7	6	8	8	2	9	4	3	0	0	0	0	0.8	4
4, RA, 35, F	5 months	1.9	0	5[e]	5[e]	3[e]	5	4	5	4	5	4	2[e]	0.3	6
5, RA, 40, M	1 yr	0.5	4	6	6	6	5	4	5	4	4	3	1	0.4	6
6, LL, 24, M	2 yr	1.4	7	8	8	8	5	5	5	0	0	0	8	1.3	Unresolved
7, LL, 38, F	3 yr	n.d.[f]	4	5	5	5	4	4	0	0	0	0	5	n.d.	Unresolved
8, LL, 27, M	2 yr	2.1	7	8	8	8	4	4	0	0	0	0	8	2.6	Unresolved

Table 1

Patient characteristics and the effect of the control and intervention phases on their pain at presentation; the frequency of mirror use on follow-up and final pain scores at 6 weeks with infra-red thermal temperature differences between affected and unaffected limbs

LA, left arm; LL, left leg; RA, right arm; F, female; M, male; n.d., not done.

[a]Region of interest constant significant difference if >0.48C;
[b]both limbs (no device);
[c]painful limb hidden;
[d]mirror visual feedback;
[e]stiffness;
[f]case 7 had widespread ulceration on her left leg, which made thermal imaging impossible.

Subject	Analgesia	IRSB (G)	Physiotherapy modalities	Occupational therapy	Immobilization	TENS	Osteopathy	Acupuncture
1	NSAID, simple		+					
2	NSAID, compound		+	+				
3	Compound		+					
4	NSAID		+				+	
5	Compound		+		+			
6	Opioid	+	+					+
7	Opioid	+	+		+	+		
8	NSAID	+	+		+			

Table 2
Therapeutic
interventions
before mirror
visual feedback

IRSB (G), intravenous regional sympathetic blockade (guanethidine);
TENS, transcutaneous electrical nerve stimulation;
NSAID, non-steroidal anti-inflammatory drug.

Subject	Analgesia	Physiotherapy modalities	Occupational therapy	Osteopathy
1	Simple	+		
2	NSAID	+	+	
3	Compound	+		
4	None	+		+
5	Compound			
6	Opioid	+		
7	Opioid	+		
8	NSAID	+		

Table 3
Treatment
received during
study protocol in
addition to mirror
visual feedback

NSAID, non-steroidal anti-inflammatory drug.

Our subjects' pain and stiffness, signalled by this incongruence, can be corrected by the use of false but nevertheless congruent visual feedback of the unaffected limb. The mirror reflection permits the subject to rehearse and practice movements of the affected limb without having to directly activate those parts of maladaptive central processes that typically produce pain. The centrally processed visual input, which appears to originate from the dysfunctional and painful side, acts to re-establish the normal pain-free relationship between sensory feedback and motor intention and consequently results in the rapid resolution of the pain state. In the absence of mirror feedback, movement exacerbates the pain, as was demonstrated in our control stages. In our subjects with long-standing disease there are two possible reasons why mirror visual feedback was ineffective. The first was that trophic changes, such as contractures, limited movement, and the second was that neural pathways may be more established over time. The effect in the two intermediate cases, in whom the easing of stiffness was more apparent than an analgesic response, provides further evidence that time plays a part in this process. Interestingly, single photon emission computed tomography studies [14] have shown that the early stages of the illness are associated with increased blood flow in the thalamus while in the later stages this region shows hypoperfusion. These changes and the peripheral changes that occur over time may explain the lack of treatment effect in subjects with chronic CRPS and the more limited effect in the intermediate cases.

Not withstanding the therapeutic implications, our results provide an important insight into the pathogenesis of CRPS and possibly other conditions presenting with 'inappropriate' pain. Larger studies, supported ideally by functional imaging, are required.

During the final preparation of this manuscript, Professor Patrick Wall died (8 August 2001) and the other authors would like to dedicate this paper to his memory.

Acknowledgments
We are grateful to the patients who assisted in this study. We thank the physicians at The Royal National Hospital for Rheumatic Diseases for allowing us to study their patients and Mr D. Elvins and Miss R. Edwards for technical assistance. This work was financed by an Arthritis Research Campaign Integrated Clinical Arthritis Centre Award. CSM is supported as an Arthritis Research Campaign Lecturer in Rheumatological Nursing. RCH is supported as an Arthritis Research Campaign Clinical Research Fellow. PWH is funded by the Medical Research Council.

Notes

Correspondence to: C. S. McCabe, The Royal National Hospital for Rheumatic Diseases, Upper Borough Walls, Bath BA1 1RL, UK.
E-mail: candy.mccabe@rnhrd-tr.swest.nhs.uk

References

1. Scadding JW. Complex regional pain syndrome. In: Wall PD, Melzack R, eds. Textbook of pain. 4th edition. Edinburgh: Churchill Livingstone, 1999:835–50.

2. Jaded AR, Carroll D, Glynn CJ, McQuay H. Intravenous regional sympathetic blockade for pain relief in reflex sympathetic dystrophy: a systematic review and a randomised, double-blind crossover study. J Pain Symptom Manage 1995;10:13–9.

3. Ramachandran VS, Roger-Ramachandran D. Synaesthesia in phantom limbs induced with mirrors. Proc R Soc Lond B Biol Sci 1996;263:377–86.

4. Melzack R, Wall PD. Pain mechanisms: a new theory. Science 1965;150:971–99.

5. Wall PD. Pain, the science of suffering. London: Weidenfeld and Nicolson, 1999.

6. Wall PD. Pain in context: The intellectual roots of pain research and therapy. Proceedings of the 9th World Congress on Pain. In: Devor M, Rowbotham MC, Wiessenfeld-Hallin Z, eds. Progress in Pain Research and Management, Vol. 16. Seattle: IASP Press, 2000, P19–33.

7. Flor H, Braun C, Elbert T, Birbaumer N. Extensive reorganization of primary somatosensory cortex in chronic back pain patients. Neurosci Lett 1997;224:5–8.

8. Byl NN, Melnick M. The neural consequences of repetition: clinical implications of a learning hypothesis. J Hand Ther 1997;10:160–74.

9. Ramachandran VS, Rogers-Ramachandran D, Stewart M. Perceptual correlates of massive cortical reorganisation. Science 1992;258:1159–60.

10. Flor H, Elbert T, Knecht S, et al. Phantom-limb pain as a perceptual correlate of cortical reorganization following arm amputation. Nature 1995;375:482–4.

11. Fink GR, Marshall JC, Halligan PW, et al. The neural consequences of conflict between intention and the senses. Brain 1999;122:497–512.

12. Harris AJ. Cortical origins of pathological pain. Lancet 1999;354:1464–6.
13. Uematsu S, Edwin DH, Jankel VVR, *et al.* Quantification of thermal asymmetry. Part 1. Normal values and reproducibility. J Neurosurg 1988;69:552–5.
14. Fukumoto M, Ushida T, Zinchuk VS, Yamamoto H, Yoshida S. Contralateral thalamic perfusion in patients with reflex sympathetic dystrophy syndrome. Lancet 1999;354:1790–1.

Submitted 20 March 2002; accepted 7 June 2002
Rheumatology 2003;42:97–101

ooooo

Phantom Limb Pain in Amputees

Vilayanur Ramachandran is Director of the Center for Brain and Cognition and Professor with the Psychology Department in the Neurosciences Program at the University of California, San Diego. He is an Adjunct Professor of Biology at the Salk Institute. Having trained as a doctor Ramachandran went on to acquire a Ph.D from Trinity College – Cambridge University. His early research was on visual perception, but he is best known for his work in behavioural neurology. Richard Dawkins called him "The Marco Polo of Neuroscience".

The following is an excerpt from 'Phantoms in the Brain' by Sandra Blakeslee and V.S. Ramachandran.
© *Harper Collins*

Here V. Ramachandran describes some work with amputees experiencing Phantom Pain.

Pain is one of the most poorly understood of all sensory experiences. It is a source of great frustration to patient and physician alike and can emerge in many different guises. One especially enigmatic complaint frequently heard from patients is that every now and again the phantom hand becomes curled into a tight, white knuckled fist, fingers digging into palm with all the fury of a prize fighter ready to deliver a knockout blow.

Robert Townsend is an intelligent, fifty-five-year-old engineer whose cancer caused him to lose his left arm six inches above the elbow. When I saw him seven months after the amputation, he was experiencing a vivid phantom limb that would often go into an involuntary clenching spasm. "Its like my nails are digging into my phantom hand," said Robert. "The pain is unbearable." Even if he concentrated all his attention on it, he could not open his invisible hand to relieve the spasm.

We wondered whether using the mirror box could help Robert eliminate his spasms. Like Philip, Robert looked into the box, positioned his good hand to superimpose its reflection over his phantom hand and, after making a fist with the normal hand, tried to unclench both hands simultaneously. The first time he did this Robert exclaimed that he could feel the phantom fist opening along with his good fist, simply as a result of the visual feedback. Better yet, the pain disappeared. The phantom then remained unclenched for several hours until a new spasm occurred spontaneously. Without the mirror, his phantom would throb in pain for forty minutes or more. Robert took the box home and tried the same trick each time that the clenching spasm recurred. If he did not use the box, he could not unclench his fist despite trying with all his might. If he used the mirror the hand opened instantly.

We have tried this treatment in over a dozen patients and it works for half of them. They take the mirrored box home and whenever a spasm occurs, they put their good hand into the box and open it and the spasm is eliminated. But is it a cure? It's difficult to know. Pain is notoriously susceptible to the placebo effect (the power of suggestion). Perhaps the elaborate laboratory setting or the mere presence of a charismatic expert on phantom limbs is all you need in order to eliminate the pain and has nothing to do with mirrors. We tested this possibility on one patient by giving him a harmless battery pack that generates an electrical current. Whenever the spasms and abnormal posture occurred he was asked to rotate the dial on the unit of his 'transcutaneous electrical stimulator' until he began to feel a tingling in his left arm (which was his good arm). We told him that this would immediately restore voluntary movements in the phantom and provide relief from the spasms. We also told him that the procedure had worked on other patients in his predicament. He said "Really? Wow, I can't wait to try it."

Two days later he was back, obviously annoyed. "It's useless," he exclaimed. "I tried it five times and it just doesn't work. I turned it up to full strength even though you told me not to."

When I gave him the mirror to try that afternoon, he was able to open his phantom hand instantly. The spasms were eliminated and so too was the 'digging sensation' of nails biting into his palm. This is a mind boggling observation if you think about it. Here is a man with no hand and no fingernails. How does one get nonexistent nails digging into a nonexistent palm, resulting in severe pain? Why would a mirror eliminate the phantom spasm?

Consider what happens in your brain when motor commands are sent from the premotor and motor cortex to make a fist. Once you hand is clenched, feedback signals from muscles and joints of your hand are sent back through the spinal chord to your brain saying, Slow down, enough. Any more pressure and it could hurt. This proprioceptive feedback applies brakes, automatically, with astonishing speed and precision.

If the limb is missing however, this damping feedback is not possible. The brain therefore keeps sending the message, Clench more, clench more, clench more. Motor output is amplified even further (to a level that far exceeds anything you or I would ever experience) and the overflow or 'sense of effort' may itself be experienced as pain. The mirror may work by providing visual feedback to unclench the hand, so that the clenching spasm is abolished.

But why the sensation of the digging fingernails? Just think of the numerous occasions when you actually clenched your fist and felt your nails biting into your palm. These occasions must have created a memory link in your brain (psychologists call it a Hebbian link) between the motor command to clench and the unmistakable sensation of 'nails digging', so you can readily summon up this image in your mind. Yet even though you can imagine the image quite vividly, you don't actually feel the sensation and say, "Ouch, that hurts." Why not? The reason, I believe, is that you have a real palm and the skin on the palm says there is no pain. You can imagine it but you don't feel it because you have a normal hand sending real feedback and in the clash between reality and illusion, reality usually wins.

But the amputee doesn't have a palm. There are no countermanding signals from the palm to forbid the emergence of these stored pain memories. When Robert imagines that his nails are digging into his hand, he doesn't get contradictory signals from his skin surface saying, "Robert, you fool, there's no pain down here." Indeed, if the motor commands themselves are linked to the sense of nail digging, it is conceivable that the amplification of these commands leads to a corresponding amplification of the associated pain signals. This might explain why the pain is so brutal.

The implications are radical. Even fleeting sensory associations such as the one between clenching our hands and digging our fingernails into our palms are laid down as permanent traces in the brain and are only unmasked under certain circumstances – experienced in this case as phantom limb pain. Moreover, these ideas imply that pain is an *opinion* on the organism's state of health rather than a mere reflexive response to an injury. There is no direct hot-line from pain receptors to 'pain centres' in the brain. On the contrary, there is so much interaction between different brain centres, like those concerned with vision and touch, that even the mere visual appearance of an opening fist can actually feed all the way back into the patient's motor and touch pathways, allowing him to feel the fist opening, thereby killing an illusory pain in a nonexistent hand.

If pain is an illusion, how much influence do senses like vision have over our subjective experiences? To find out, I tried a somewhat diabolical experiment on two of my patients. When Mary came into the lab, I asked her to place her phantom right hand, palm down into the mirror box. I then asked her to put a gray glove on her good left hand and place it in the other side of the box, in a mirror image position. After making sure she was comfortable I instructed one of my graduate students to hide under the curtained table and put his gloved hand into the same side of the box where Mary's good hand rested, above hers on a false platform. When Mary looked into the box she could see not only the student's gloved left hand (which looked exactly like her own left hand) but also its reflection in the mirror, as if she were looking at her own phantom right hand wearing a glove. When the student now made a fist or used his index finger to touch the ball of his thumb, Mary felt her phantom moving vividly. As in our previous two patients, vision was enough to trick her brain into experiencing movements in her phantom limb.

What would happen if we fooled Mary into thinking that her fingers were occupying anatomically impossible positions? The box permitted this illusion. Again, Mary put her phantom right hand, palm down, in the box. But the student now did something different. Instead of placing his left hand into the other side of the box, in an exact mirror image of the phantom, he inserted his right hand, palm up. Since the hand was gloved, it looked exactly like her 'palm down' phantom right hand. Then the student flexed his index finger to touch his palm. To Mary, peering into the box, it appeared as if her phantom index finger were bending backward to touch the back of her wrist! What would her reaction be?

When Mary saw her finger twisted backward, she said, "One would have thought it should feel peculiar, doctor, but it doesn't. It feels exactly like the finger is bending backward, like it isn't supposed to. But it doesn't feel peculiar or painful or anything like that."

Another subject, Karen, winced and said that the twisted phantom finger hurt. "It felt like somebody was grabbing and pulling my finger. I felt a twinge of pain," she said.

These experiments are important because they flatly contradict the theory that the brain consists of a number of autonomous modules acting as a bucket brigade. Popularised by artificial intelligence researchers, the idea that the brain behaves like a computer, with each module performing a highly specialised job and sending its output to the next module, is widely believed. In this view, sensory processing involves a one-way cascade of information sensory receptors on the skin and other sense organs to higher brain centres.

But my experiments with these patients have taught me that this is not how the brain works. Its connections are extraordinarily labile and dynamic. Perceptions emerge as a result of reverberations of signals between different levels of the sensory hierarchy, indeed even across different senses. The fact that visual input can eliminate the spasm of a nonexistent arm and then erase the associated memory of pain vividly illustrates how extensive and profound these interactions can be.

Reprinted by Permission Harper Collins Ltd.
© *V.S. Ramachandran and Sandra Blakeslee* 1998

V.S. Ramachandran Delivered the Reith Lecture 2003
www.bbc.co.uk/radio4/reith2003/

He can also be seen on:
www.ted.com/speakers/vilayanur_ramachandran.html

Phantoms in the Brain – Published by Harper Collins
ISBN 978-1-85702-895-9

Manual of Contacts

Pain Relief Foundation

A Unique Medical Charity

In 1979, three doctors working in the Walton Centre in Liverpool, Dr. Sam Lipton, Professor John Miles and Dr. David Bowsher, realised that in treating their patients, they were dealing with the same largely unsolved problems of chronic pain. Then they discovered that there was no existing research for investigating human chronic pain because there was no funding from the NHS, the Government or any Public organization for this work. Therefore, they decided to setup their own Charity – The Pain Relief Foundation, with the twin functions of research and teaching Health Professionals how to use the results of the research, in treating chronic pain patients.

The Foundation opened a Pain Research Institute in Liverpool because in Liverpool, the Walton Centre Pain Clinic had a huge number of chronic pain patients. It was the first, and today remains the *only* Research Institute of its kind devoted entirely to multidisciplinary research on human chronic pain and it is here that we work on these conditions. Importantly, animals are not used in experiments at the Pain Research Institute.

The wide-ranging research programmes use many different techniques to investigate the causes and alleviation of the many types of chronic pain: neuropathic pain, facial pain, post-stroke pain, neuralgia pain, migraine and severe headaches, diabetic pain, shingles and many other categories, each of which are very severe pain conditions; all non-fatal, but which bring with them a life sentence of misery and despair.

Consider also phantom limb pain (the limb has been amputated, but severe pain is still coming from that area of the body). These problems are difficult to explain, not easy for many to understand, particularly as most normal pain can be controlled by a course of 'over-the-counter medicines' such as paracetamol, aspirin, codeine or ibuprofen. But chronic pain cannot be controlled in this way.

So you can understand why our work on helping to relieve the pain suffered by cancer patients, for instance, is vital. Many cancer charities and research organisations are unable to fund research work on cancer pain because their trust deeds specify 'research into the cause and cure of cancer' but *not* into the **relief of pain in cancer**. Therefore, our work in pain associated with this disease is very important. Over the years there have been a vast number of very significant breakthroughs. For instance, over time some cancer patients become inured to the pain-relieving benefits of morphine. Research into this problem in the Foundation's laboratories discovered that pain relief could be restored by changing to other opiate-based drugs, bringing the patient peace and dignity at that ultimate difficult time in their illness. Yet for every £1.57 that is donated to cancer research, chronic pain research receives *less* than **one penny**.

Scientists and medical specialists from all over the world go to the Pain Research Institute as visiting researchers. They stay as long as one or even two years working on all types of human chronic pain alongside the Foundation's permanent staff. Already there are many thousands of patients world-wide who are benefiting from the many treatments which have been pioneered at the Pain Research Institute.

The Pain Research Institute has developed a truly important educational role. That is why we also conduct educational courses for health professionals at all levels, providing them with the knowledge about new and emerging methods of recognising and treating chronic pain conditions, and this includes surgical techniques, across the many health disciplines. In fact, many of the doctors working in Pain Clinics across the UK have received much of their training at the Institute and the clinic with which it is associated.

The fight against human chronic pain is one of the last great challenges facing medical science and perhaps you may wish to help the Pain Relief Foundation with their work to relieve the suffering of others by making a donation to their funds.

Chronic Pain doesn't kill; it just causes a life-sentence of never ending misery and suffering. No matter how much you treat the pain it doesn't go away; strong painkilling drugs often don't work; the pain is relentless and sufferers lead a lifetime of agony!

If you wish to make a donation, or if you need any help or any information leaflets from the Pain Relief Foundation, they can be contacted at:

The Pain Relief Foundation
Clinical Sciences Centre
University Hospital Aintree   Tel: 0151 529 5820
Liverpool L9 7AL   Fax: 0151 529 5821
United Kingdom   secretary@painrelieffoundation.org.uk

www.painrelieffoundation.org.uk

ooooo

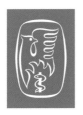

British Association of Occupational Therapists and College of Occupational Therapists

The Occupational Therapist Role

Occupational therapists are health and social care professionals who help people of all ages – babies, children, adults and older people – to carry out activities they need or want to do, but as a result of physical or mental illness, disability or being socially excluded, they are prevented from doing the activities they value. These could include the everyday necessities of daily living, such as preparing a meal, or getting dressed, going to school or work, or simply continuing with a favourite hobby. They could be more complex activities such as caring for children, succeeding in studies or work, or maintaining a healthy social life. Occupational therapists will work with individuals to find alternative ways to do those activities to help people live their life their way.

Occupational therapy has a unique philosophy that acknowledges the link between what people do and their health and wellbeing. To the profession 'occupation' means all the activities a person undertakes, enjoys and values. More importantly, everything we do – our daily occupations – help to define our identity and role. If an individual is unable to do what is important to them and fulfil their role, their health and wellbeing can suffer. Occupational therapists can address this by enabling individuals to find ways to do those activities that are important to them.

An occupational therapists work could involve:
- Making sure that homes workplaces and public places are accessible for people with specific needs, for example wheelchair users or people with walking difficulties or partial sight.
- Helping people to learn new or different ways of doing things, for example how do you think you would turn over this page if you couldn't use your hands?
- Adapting materials or equipment, for example what might you suggest if a computer keyboard was difficult to use?
- Advising in schools to help children overcome obstacles such as writing difficulties and other learning challenges.

- Heading up a disability management programme for an organisation, or return-to-work programmes for people with anxiety or back problems.
- Assisting an ageing couple to care for one another in their own home and remain independent and safe.
- Helping someone manage their depression in order to return to work or continue with their studies.
- Setting up a rehabilitation programme in a developing or war-torn region.
- Working with socially excluded groups, such as the homeless or asylum seekers.

Further information about occupational therapy is available from the College of Occupational Therapists website: **www.cot.org.uk**

College of Occupational Therapists
106–114 Borough High Street
Southwark
London SE1 1LB
United Kingdom   Tel: 020 7357 6480

CRPS and Occupational Therapy
Assessment by an occupational therapist with skills in the treatment of Complex Regional Pain Syndrome (CRPS) is recommended for anyone living with this condition. The aim of occupational therapy treatment is to restore as much quality of life as possible and to try and give some control over CRPS symptoms. The occupational therapist will help to find ways of being able to manage everyday activities at home and work, and to improve access to interests, hobbies and sports. It may not be possible to change the level of pain greatly.

A variety of techniques can be used to improve function and help manage pain.

These include:
Desensitisation – a treatment that aims to restore normal feeling to the affected skin area. This involves frequently touching the skin with a range of textures, gradually working into the most painful areas.

Restoration of a normal body image – some people find it difficult or distressing to look at the area affected by CRPS or are unsure of where their affected arm or leg is without looking at it. The occupational therapist can teach relaxation and visualisation strategies to help overcome this.

Pacing – an effective method of being able to manage daily routines without intensifying pain levels and causing fatigue. Pacing includes developing relaxation skills to manage pain and anxiety, addressing poor sleep habits, setting goals and making suggestions on how to increase overall fitness levels.

Hand Therapy – the use of appropriate exercises and the use of media such as warm wax to increase the range of movement and grip strength of a person whose hand is affected by CRPS.

Equipment Advice – the selection of small aids to complete everyday activities such as dressing, meal preparation or writing. If walking sticks or elbow crutches are used, the occupational therapist will help to find safer, easier ways to carry items.

The occupational therapist may also recommend other treatment approaches dependent on individual circumstances and can work with other agencies, such as local councils or employers, when appropriate.

With thanks to author of Occupational Therapy and CRPS:
Karen Coales, Senior Occupational Therapist – Rheumatology
Royal National Hospital for Rheumatic Diseases. Bath

📖 **For Royal National Hospital Rheumatic Diseases CRPS Service see page 198**

📖 **For information on the history of Occupational Therapy see page 226**

ooooo

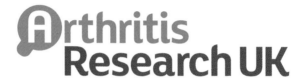

Providing answers today and tomorrow

Arthritis Research UK is the charity leading the fight against arthritis.

We're working to take the pain away for sufferers of all forms of arthritis and helping people to remain active. We do this by funding high class research, providing information and campaigning.

Everything we do is underpinned by research.

Our Vision
Our vision is a future free from arthritis.

Our Mission
Our mission is to reduce the pain and disability resulting from arthritis by:
- funding high quality research into the cause, treatment and cure of arthritis and translating the results of that research to benefit patients
- educating and informing the general public, patients and health professionals on all aspects of arthritis
- campaigning for better treatment and support for all those living with arthritis
- working in partnership with others to make a greater difference for people with arthritis.

We produce more than 90 patient information booklets and online publications for patients on all types of arthritis and musculoskeletal conditions, including complex regional pain syndrome (also known as reflex sympathetic dystrophy) available at **www.arthritisresearchuk.org**

To request one of our 90 booklets please phone 01904 696994.

We are funding research into the painful condition of complex regional pain syndrome at research centres in Bath and in Salford, with the aim of improving treatment of this little-understood condition.

Arthritis Research UK
St Mary's Gate
Chesterfield
Derbyshire
S41 7TD
United Kingdom

Tel: +44 (0) 1246 558033
Fax: +44 (0) 1246 558007
enquiries@arthritisresearchuk.org

ooooo

CRPS Service
Royal National Hospital for Rheumatic Diseases NHS Foundation Trust

Upper Borough Walls
Bath
BA1 1RL
United Kingdom

Tel: 01225 465941
info@rnhrd.nhs.uk

www.rnhrd.nhs.uk

ooooo

The British Association of Hand Therapists (BAHT) is an association of Physiotherapists and Occupational Therapists who specialise in the treatment of conditions of the hand. BAHT is a specialist clinical interest group of the Chartered Society of Physiotherapy (CSP).
Information about the British Association of Hand Therapists and hand therapy can be found on their website **www.hand-therapy.co.uk**

Tel: 01394 610131

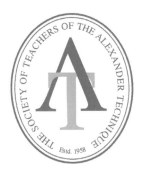

*The oldest and largest professional society
of teachers of the Alexander Technique*

Regain Control of your Body to Alleviate Pain,
Improve Posture and Enhance Performance

*"You feel an amazing lightness, like you've been suddenly
given the body of someone ten years younger"*

STAT pupil survey 2006

The Alexander Technique works by helping you to identify and prevent the harmful postural habits that aggravate, or may be the cause of, stress, pain, and under-performance.

You will learn how to release tension and rediscover balance of mind and body. With increased awareness you can:
- be poised without stiffness
- move gracefully and powerfully with less effort
- be alert and focussed with less strain
- breathe and speak more easily and freely
- be calm and confident

Learning the Alexander Technique can help to prevent or alleviate conditions associated with undue tension or poor posture. These include many difficulties with pain and weakness, co-ordination and movement, and joint or muscle problems. Examining the way people carry themselves and hold tension, and teaching them to move more naturally and freely, can address the underlying cause of many such problems.

The Alexander Technique can enhance rehabilitation after surgery, injury, or illness. It can improve management of pain and provide coping skills for chronic illness and disabilities.

© The Society of Teachers of the Alexander Technique. STAT

Contact the STAT Office
Opening times: 10.00 AM to 5.00 PM, Monday to Friday

The Society of Teachers of the Alexander Technique
1st Floor, Linton House
39–51 Highgate Road   Tel: 0207 482 5135
London NW5 1RS   Fax: 0207 482 5435
United Kingdom   office@stat.org.uk

www.stat.org.uk

📖 **For information on the history of Alexander Technique see page 229**

ooooo

AN OLD CURE FOR A MODERN MALAISE: ALEXANDER TECHNIQUE CAN BEAT CHRONIC BACK PAIN
By Jenny Hope Daily Mail – 20th August 2008

Back pain costs the UK economy five billion pounds each year in lost working days.

A method of relaxation developed more than 100 years ago can help ease chronic back pain, researchers say.

The Alexander Technique, formulated by an Australian actor after he lost his voice, has been proved to be effective in clinical trials.

The discovery could help British firms save vast sums of money. Each year back pain accounts for up to five million lost working days, and costs the economy an estimated five billion pounds.

A study of almost 600 patients suffering chronic or recurrent back pain found significant improvements after a year among those having lessons in the Alexander Technique.

They spent just three days in pain each month, compared with 21 days for those getting normal NHS care.

And a short course of six lessons, combined with exercise, produced almost as much benefit as a full regime of 24.

This is the first long-term study of its kind into the technique, which was originally devised to help its founder, actor Frederick Matthias Alexander, get over losing his voice during recitals.

He believed his problem was caused by the way he stiffened his whole body as he prepared to speak.

The technique has been taught in the UK since 1904, but until now there has been no thorough investigation into its long-term effectiveness and doctors have complained of the lack of evidence to support it.

Its aim is to make people more aware of how they use their bodies, and to get them to stop bad habits and excessive muscular tension.

In the latest study, published online in the British Medical Journal, a team from Southampton and Bristol Universities recruited 579 patients with chronic or recurring back pain from 64 GP areas in the south and west of England.

They were allocated one of four types of treatment – normal care such as pain-killers, physiotherapy or GP referral, massage, six Alexander technique lessons, or 24 AT lessons.

Half of the patients from each group were also prescribed an exercise programme, consisting of brisk walking for 30 minutes a day five times a week.

The £750,000 study, partly funded by the NHS, showed that lessons in the technique provided an individualised approach to reducing back pain. Participants were taught on a one-to-one basis. They learned to sit, stand and move correctly, and they also worked on their posture.

All the patients involved in the study were sent questionnaires after three months and one year asking which everyday activities were limited by their back pain.

After a year, the researchers found that exercise combined with AT lessons significantly reduced pain and improved functioning, while massage offered little benefit after three months.

Those having AT lessons also reported fewer days with back pain over the previous four weeks.

Patients getting normal care had 21 days of back pain, compared with four among those having a full 24-lesson course of the Alexander Technique. Those who had six lessons had 11 days of pain and those having massage had 14.

Co-author Professor Paul Little of the University of Southampton said: "This is a significant step forward in the long-term management of low back pain." The results of this study revealed that the Alexander Technique can help back pain.

'It probably does this by limiting muscle spasm, strengthening postural muscles, improving coordination and flexibility and decompressing the spine.'

© *Daily Mail*

ooooo

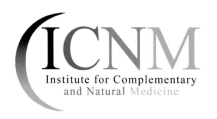

The Institute for Complementary and Natural Medicine – the Voice of Complementary Medicine

The Institute for Complementary and Natural Medicine (ICNM) provides the public with information on all aspects of the safe and best practice of Complementary Medicine through its practitioners, courses and research. It also strives to build a bridge between complementary and natural medicine and allopathic healthcare.

The ICNM's mission is to support the educational development and growth of the CAM profession whilst safeguarding the public.

The ICNM believes that the key to providing patients with the best possible care, there should be continued integration between complementary and conventional medicine.

One of the most important functions of the ICNM is administering the British Register of Complementary Practitioners (BRCP) which is a register of professional Practitioners and Therapists who have provided evidence of their individual competence to practice.

The BRCP was launched in 1989, making it one of the longest-running Registers of its kind in the country. It is a multi-disciplinary Register containing some 25 Divisions, representing about 100 different types of complementary practices. Its Members range from Acupuncturists to Aromatherapists, Hypnotherapists and Reflexologists, to name a few. In order to qualify to be a member of the BRCP, practitioners must prove their competence to practice by either completing an approved course or through an assessment made by the BRCP Registration Panel. The ICNM and BRCP are committed to ensuring the highest standards of training and continued professional development which means that, if a member of the public consults a BRCP Member, they can be confident the Practitioner is trained to the highest level of competence and are also insured.

The term complementary and alternative medicine refers to any therapy that is not provided by orthodox health professionals like doctors, nurses and dentists, although many orthodox health professionals have also trained in complementary medicine in order to provide an integrated service.

Contact details:
The Institute for Complementary and Natural Medicine
Can-Mezzanine
32–36 Loman Street   Tel: 0207 922 7980
London SE1 0EH   Fax: 0207 922 7981

www.icnm.org.uk

ooooo

THE NATIONAL INSTITUTE
OF MEDICAL
HERBALISTS

What is Herbal Medicine?

Herbal Medicine is the use of plant remedies in the treatment of disease. It is the oldest form of medicine known.

Our ancestors by trial and error, found the most effective local plants to heal their illnesses. Now with the advancement of science enabling us to identify the chemical constituents within these plants, we can better understand their healing powers.

Herbalism in this country is now classed as an 'alternative' or 'complementary' discipline, but it is still the most widely practised form of medicine worldwide with over 80% of the world's population relying on herbs for health.

The Herbalist's Approach

Medical Herbalists are trained in the same diagnostic skills as orthodox doctors, but take a more holistic approach to illness. The underlying cause of the problem is sought and once identified it is *this* which is treated, rather than the symptoms alone. The reason for this is that the treatment or suppression of symptoms will not rid the body of the disease itself. Herbalists use their medicines to restore the balance of the body, thus enabling it to mobilise its own healing powers.

The first consultation will generally take at least an hour. The Herbalist will take notes on the patient's medical history and begin to build a picture of the person as a whole being. Healing is a matter of teamwork with patient, practitioner and the prescribed treatment, all working together to restore the body to health.

Treatment may include advice about diet and lifestyle as well as the herbal medicine.

The second appointment may follow in two weeks, subsequent ones occurring monthly – this will depend on the individual herbalist, the patient and the illness concerned.

How do herbs work?

People have always relied on plants for food to nourish and sustain the body. Herbal medicine can be seen in the same way. Plants with a particular affinity for certain organs or systems of the body are used to 'feed' and restore to health those parts which have become weakened. As the body is strengthened, so is its power and ability to fight off disease and when balance and harmony are restored, health will be regained.

What are the Differences between Pharmaceutical and Herbal drugs?

Many of the pharmaceutical drugs used today are based on plant constituents and even now, when scientists are seeking new 'cures' for disease, it is to the plant world that they turn. They find, extract and then synthesise in the laboratory a single active constituent from the plant (the active constituent is the part of the plant that has the therapeutic value) and this can be manufactured on a large scale.

Herbal drugs, however, are extracts from a part of the whole plant (e.g. leaves, roots, berries etc.) and contain hundreds, perhaps thousands of plant constituents. Herbalists believe that the active constituents are balanced within the plant and are made more (or less) powerful by the numerous other substances present. For example the herb Ephedra sinica is the source of the alkaloid ephedrine which is used, in orthodox medicine, to treat asthma and nasal congestion, but it has the side effect of raising blood pressure. Within the whole plant there are six other alkaloids, one of which prevents a rise in blood pressure. Synthetic diuretics (drugs that increase the flow of urine) seriously reduce the potassium level in the body this has to be restored using potassium supplements. The Herbalist uses Dandelion leaves which are a potent diuretic but contain potassium to naturally replace that which is lost.

What can Herbal Medicine Treat?

Herbal medicine can treat almost any condition that patients might take to their doctor. Common complaints seen by herbalists include skin problems such as psoriasis, acne and eczema, digestive disorders such as peptic ulcers, colitis, irritable bowel syndrome and indigestion. Problems involving the heart and circulation like angina, high blood pressure, varicose veins, varicose ulcers etc. can also be treated successfully as can gynaecological disorders like premenstrual syndrome and menopausal problems. Also conditions such as arthritis, insomnia, stress, migraine and headaches, tonsillitis, influenza and allergic responses like hayfever and asthma. Qualified herbalists know when a condition is best seen by a doctor or another therapist.

For further details or a Register of qualified Members send a large stamped addressed envelope with postage to cover 150 g weight to:

The National Institute of Medical Herbalists
Elm House. 54 St Mary Arches Street   Tel: +44 (0) 1392 426 022
Exeter EX4 3BA   Fax +44 (0) 1392 498 963
United Kingdom   info@nimh.org.uk

www.nimh.org.uk

ooooo

It is important to be very clear about a decision to use any of the therapies discussed in this book. They are included because they worked for me and in the hope that they will stimulate an interest in more holistic approaches to pain, but not intended to replace consultation with a GP.

OSTEOPATHY

Osteopathy is a form of hands-on treatment that is suitable for people of all ages and in any state of health. It is much more than just manipulative treatment for back pain; the art of manipulating joints is an ancient one, but Osteopathy as envisaged by its founder, Andrew Taylor Still, has much greater scope and depth.

Origins
In the late 19th century Dr. Still, a country doctor in Midwest America, observed that the body's structure was reciprocally related to the way it functioned. He found that freedom of motion of all parts of the body – ensuring that fluids can interchange freely through every tissue and organ – was fundamental to its health. His particular interest was in the spine, as the 'junction box' for the neural control of the organs, muscles, circulation and all tissues.

Unique Approach to Treatment
The Osteopath works to gently realign the spinal and peripheral joints and the fascial compartments enveloping each organ, nerve, muscle and bone, to enable integrated healthy motion of the body as a whole. Osteopathy is much more than a system of techniques; true Osteopathy, as taught by Dr. Still, consists of the 'osteopathic thinking' used in understanding the route by which the problem came into being, which also indicates the way in which the body needs to be treated to unlock its own self-healing potential.

General Osteopathic Council
176 Tower Bridge Road
London SE1 3LU
United Kingdom

Tel: +44 (0) 20 7357 6655
Fax: +44 (0) 20 7357 0011
contactus@osteopathy.org.uk

www.osteopathy.org.uk

📖 **For information on the history of Osteopathy see page 233**

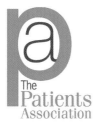

The Patients Association is a national charity providing patients with an opportunity to raise concerns and share experiences of healthcare.

Through our Helpline, correspondence and research we learn from patients the issues that are of concern and work towards improving the healthcare we all receive.

The Patients Association was set up more than 40 years ago to promote the voice of patients in healthcare. We are a registered charity based in North London staffed by paid and unpaid staff committed to making a difference to the 'Patient Journey'.

We offer patients an opportunity to share their experiences of health services and use the knowledge gained from patients to work with the NHS and other healthcare providers in improving services.

Working with a range of organisations providing health services we receive income through individual members, corporate members in the commercial sector, specific project work, consultations and events. We are an entirely independent organisation and *do not* receive any core organisation funding from the Department of Health or any other government body.

For more information about the association and the work we carry out please explore our site. The Patients Association's charity number is 1006733.

If you would like to become an E-Member of the Patients Association for free, simply go to our homepage, enter your email address and you will receive a copy of our free weekly news round up.

If you would like to become a member, please send us an email to mailbox@patients-association.com. We will shortly provide you with full information on how to get more involved on the Patients Association activities.

For those who require membership and newsletters in hard copy please call 020 8423 9111.

To contact the Patients Association's administration office, including press officers:

The Patients Association
PO Box 935
Harrow, Middlesex
HAI 3YJ
United Kingdom

Tel: 020 8423 9111
Fax: 020 8423 9119
Helpline: 0845 608 4455
helpline@patients-association.com

www.patients-association.com

ooooo

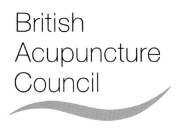

British Acupuncture Council

Acupuncture has been used in China and other eastern cultures to restore, promote and maintain good health for over 2,500 years. The spread of Acupuncture knowledge has resulted in centuries of accumulated recorded experience. These sources provide the foundation for traditional Acupuncture practice today. Traditional Acupuncture takes a holistic approach to health and regards illness as a sign that the body is out of balance. The exact pattern and degree of disharmony is unique to each individual. The traditional Acupuncturist's skill lies in identifying the underlying pattern of disharmony and selecting the most effective treatment. Traditional Acupuncture can help resolve specific symptoms or conditions. It can also be used as a preventive measure to strengthen the constitution and promote general wellbeing. The choice of Acupuncture points will be specific to a patient's needs, and the needles are left in for varying lengths of time. In conjunction with needling, the practitioner may use other techniques such as moxibustion, cupping and electro-acupuncture.

The British Acupuncture Council (BAcC) was formed in 1995. With nearly 3,000 qualified members it represents the largest body of professional Acupuncturists in the UK and guarantees excellence in the following areas:

- **training**: entry to the profession is at three-year undergraduate degree level training
- **safe practice**: standards are drawn up in consultation with internationally renowned experts
- **professional conduct**: members agree to adhere to strict codes of ethics and professional conduct.

Over the past decade the British Acupuncture Council has been a key player in driving the move towards the statutory regulation of Acupuncture. Until regulation is enacted, the Council continues in its commitment to protecting both the public and its members by ensuring high standards of training, continuing education, and safe practice.

To find a qualified Acupuncturist, contact the British Acupuncture Council on 020 8735 0400 or visit **www.acupuncture.org.uk**

Collateral Meridian Therapy – Enrac

Healing the pain, one doctor at a time.

Collateral Meridian Therapy (CMT), also known as Ko Medicine, is a non-invasive acupressure technique developed by Dr. Shan-Chi Ko, who formulated a mathematical model of 108 acupoints within the 12 collateral meridians essential for alleviating various degenerative symptoms of neurological origin. Traditional Acupuncture utilizes a needle inserted into a single acupoint along one meridian to relieve the obstruction of the vital flow, while CMT manipulates two precisely defined acupoints along two different collateral meridians – one for interconnecting the diseased meridian to the treatment meridian and the other for the treatment of the diseased point in order to bypass the obstruction and restore the body's vital flow.

Ko Medicine defines vital flow as the elements, such as neurons, electrons, air, blood, lymph, and other bodily fluids, that regulate the flow of bodily energy through multiple conduits. Obstructions to vital flow can be measured with a neurometer. Removing the obstructions to vital flow not only relieves pain, but also assists in correcting abnormalities within the internal organs.

CMT is mathematical, logical, and easy to learn. No background in Acupuncture is required. CMT has been clinically applied to treat various pain and degenerative symptoms such as sports injuries, frozen shoulders, carpal tunnel syndrome, migraine headache, diabetes, fibromyalgia, PHN, and RSD/CRPS [1, 2].

For a information DVD with 18 treatment examples, request or download from the website: Enrac Europe **www.ecmt.info**

Taiwan:
Enrac Medical Society of Japan,
Taiwan Office
Tel: +886 2 2313 1200
Fax: +886 2 2313 1123
info.tw@enrac.com

Japan:
Painless Ginza Clinic
Tel: +81 3 5537 1270
info@painless-clinic.com
www.painless-clinic.com

ooooo

Conditions associated with CRPS and Other Pain Syndromes
and
Treatment Protocols

Please note there is a difference in spelling: Oedema – uk, Edema – us.

Edema

Edema – an accumulation of fluid in the body tissues that can be generalized (throughout the body) or localized (specific to one part of the body). This condition can be caused by trauma to any part of the body, or by infections, medical conditions, and autoimmune diseases. Edema can interfere with wound healing and increase the risk of infection. It can decrease joint mobility and sometimes lead to permanent loss of motion. Edema decreases blood flow in the arteries, veins and lymphatic system. Any medical condition that causes edema should be monitored by a physician. This article will focus on edema that occurs in the extremities (arms and legs).

There are several different types of edema that may occur in the extremities.

Acute

- Occurs immediately following an injury.
- Occurs as an inflammatory response to infection.

Dependent

- Occurs as the result of increased pressure in the arteries and decreased pressure in the veins, resulting in uneven fluid distribution (in any body part below the level of the heart).
- Occurs if there is a lack of muscle tone necessary to help pump blood out of the arms or legs (i.e. if there is weakness in the muscles).
- Usually affects the legs more than the arms.

Fibrotic

- Occurs when edema has been present for an extended period of time.
- Characterised by 'pitting' of the skin (when pressed with a finger, an indentation will remain).

External
- Results from an artificial cause such as a tight garment which can interfere with blood flow or lymphatic flow.

Treatment Possibilities

The most common treatment for edema is elevation of the affected body part. Other treatments may include rest, active range of motion (AROM) exercise, electromodalities, thermal modalities, medication, splinting and casting. Typically these treatments are combined to provide the quickest and most efficient reduction of the edema. You should follow the guidelines provided by a medical professional.

Tips for Managing Edema at Home

Rest is important immediately following an injury. Remember to balance rest and exercise at the beginning of your rehabilitation process. Elevation is the most effective treatment for edema. The goal is to position your arm or leg above the level of the heart.

Elevation Suggestions for the Upper Extremities
- Use pillows to raise your arm or hand when sitting or lying in bed.
- If wearing a sling, elevate your hand above the elbow.
- Place your arm on the back of the sofa when sitting.

Elevation Suggestions for the Lower Extremities
- Prop your feet up on a stool when sitting.
- Use a reclining chair to elevate your legs.
- Use pillows to raise you feet in bed.

Retrograde massage can help push fluid out of an extremity. Always massage toward your body (i.e. from fingertips toward the elbow). Use a milking technique and a moderate amount of pressure. It also helps to elevate the part being massaged. It's a good idea to use lotion or oil to lubricate the skin for the massage.

Sometimes skin can be more fragile when edema is present, so remember to inspect your skin daily for redness, blisters and breaks in the skin.

Ice can reduce edema, especially in the first 24–48 hours following an injury. Use an ice pack for 10–30 minutes several times a day over the swollen area. Check your skin carefully for hypersensitivity to ice during the treatment. Place a towel between the ice pack and your skin for extra protection.

Exercise can help pump fluid out of the extremities. Bend and straighten all of the joints of the swollen extremity. Bend and straighten 10 times for each joint. Do this every two hours or several times each day.

Author: Amy Wright, OTR

ooooo

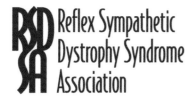

Reflex Sympathetic
Dystrophy Syndrome
Association

Raising Awareness of Complex
Regional Pain Syndrome since 1984.

The following article on Treatment Protocols for CRPS and Osteoporosis are used here by kind permission of RSDSA.

To view the full texts on their website **www.rsds.org**
This is an Organisation based in USA.

Treatment protocols

Treatment objectives for CRPS are to minimize edema, normalise sensation, promote normal positioning, decrease muscle guarding and increase independence in all areas – mobility, work, leisure and activities of daily living (ADL).

Active weight bearing exercises are emphasised.

Edema is managed using specialised garments – edema gloves etc and manual mobilisation techniques [1]. Stress loading and active range of motion (AROM) activities are also fundamental in managing edema. Elevation of the extremity can be effective; however it can sometimes become part of a cycle of guarding and disuse.

Desensitisation techniques are implemented to assist with normalising sensation to the affected area. This consists of progressive stimulation with very soft material to more textured fabrics or materials. Stimulation can be graded from light touch to deep pressure and from consistent to intermittent with each material. Contrast baths that gradually broaden the temperature difference between the two can work toward tolerance of heat or cold [1].

Posture is an important component to consider in treating CRPS. Proper posture and alignment can minimise protective guarding of the extremity, promote balanced use of muscles and facilitate improved functional use of the affected extremity.

Stress Loading consists of two principles:

Scrubbing and carrying. A stress loading programme promotes active movement and compression of the affected joints for a minimum of 3–5 consecutive minutes, three or more times each day. Though stress loading may initially produce an increase in pain or swelling of the extremity, after several days a decrease in symptoms will begin to be evident. Use of the affected extremity in daily tasks is encouraged throughout rehabilitation to inhibit muscle guarding and disuse atrophy [2, 4, 5].

Scrubbing consists of moving the affected extremity in a back/forth motion while weight bearing through the extremity [4, 5]. The patient scrubs against a hard surface, keeping the bristles of the brush in constant contact with the surface, while maintaining constant pressure on the brush. The amount of weight placed through the affected extremity and the duration of the activity are gradually increased. Scrubbing is performed with the patient in quadruped for upper extremity involvement and in elevated sitting or standing for lower extremity involvement [2].

Carrying or loading is the second component in the stress loading protocol. Small objects are carried in the hand on the affected side, progressing to a handled bag loaded with increasingly heavier weight. Carrying should be performed throughout the day, whenever the patient is standing or walking [4, 5].

Treatment summary

The overall role of the therapist during rehabilitation of CRPS is to guide the patient through a programme designed to minimise pain and edema while maximising functional use of the extremity. As CRPS varies greatly in severity and duration, it is very important for the therapist to demonstrate enthusiasm, support and encouragement of the patient during the treatment process.

The patient, in turn, must be actively involved in integration of treatment techniques into all daily activities to achieve optimal function of the affected extremity.

Author: Melanie Swan, OTR/L

References

1. Barthel J, Costa B, King A, Swan M, Harden RN. Treatment of CRPS: Functional Restoration. Submitted Clin J Pain 2002
2. Phillips ME. OT treatment for complex regional pain syndrome. OT Practt August 20, 2001.
3. Phillips ME, Katz J, Harden RN. Occupational and block therapies for complex regional pain syndrome. Paper presented at: Midwest Pain Society – AOTA National Conference, 2000; Seattle, WA
4. Carlson LK, Watson HK. Treatment of reflex sympathetic dystrophy using the stress-loading program. J Hand Ther 1988; 1: 149–54
5. Watson HK, Carlson L. Treatment of reflex sympathetic dystrophy of the hand with an active 'stress loading' program. J Hand Surg 1987; 12A (5): 779–85

ooooo

Osteoporosis
Bone Up on Osteoporosis by kind permission of RSDSA.

You can manage some of the risk of developing this degenerative bone disease
Author: Amie King

People who have complex regional pain syndrome (CRPS) should know about their increased risk for osteoporosis, a condition characterized by decreased bone mass and deterioration of bone tissue. Osteoporosis, which causes bones to become fragile and creates an increased risk for fracture, can be a concern in the dystrophic, ischemic, and atrophic stages of CRPS. Though you cannot consciously control the CRPS disease process, you can influence many of the following factors that increase the risk of developing osteoporosis.

Learned disuse
Many people with CRPS naturally, though mistakenly, avoid movements that hurt. This can lead to a 'learned disuse' pattern, which can result in bone loss and decreased tissue strength. A bone needs consistent stress placed upon it to be strong, and that stress occurs with weight bearing or when muscles pull on the bone to create movement. Because these two activities often hurt people

with CRPS, many avoid putting weight through their affected extremity, and/or using it in a normal way. For example, you might hold your hand in a guarded fashion, or use an assistive device, such as a cane or crutches. These activities decrease pain at the time, or protect the area; however, if this becomes habitual, the bone will not get the stress it needs to maintain its bone mineral density. As the bone itself weakens, the extremity's tolerance to the very activities it needs to perform to gain density weakens as well.

The importance of aerobic, weight bearing, and resistance exercises ca not be overstated. A therapist will be able to guide you through exercises and activities designed specifically to maintain functional use of your extremity as well as a healthy bone density. The goal is to create an exercise plan that achieves the right amount of stress to the bones and soft tissues of the extremity without overdoing it. A trained therapist will know what activities to initiate. Sometimes just simple active movement is all that is tolerated. This can be beneficial by providing muscular pull against the bone, which causes it to rebuild and become denser. In other circumstances, active range of motion may be contraindicated for a period of time. In these instances, a protocol involving scrubbing and carrying to stress the bone tissue without any joint motion would be better advised. Open communication with the therapists is crucial in determining the right treatment plan. Once an appropriate exercise program is designed, regular, independent completion of that program is vital. Increased activity initially may be uncomfortable, or even 'flare up' pain, but consistent diligence with the program will prove valuable over time in function, health, and pain levels.

Nutrition and Lifestyle
Everyone knows "milk does a body good", and calcium certainly is important in bone health, though there are many other factors at play. A diet rich in calcium, magnesium, vitamin D, zinc, copper, and manganese has been associated with greater bone density.

Additionally, diets too high in sodium or protein can have adverse effects on bone health. It is important to be aware that what you eat can make a substantial difference in many aspects of your health. For more specific information on the role of nutrition, speak to your doctor or a registered dietician.

Finally, cigarette smoking, excessive alcohol, and excessive caffeine have been well documented in their detrimental effects on bone density and bone health. Making changes in these areas will have positive effects on your overall health, as well as the disease process of CRPS.

In conclusion, participating in the right amount of activity and exercise is the most helpful and specific intervention to reduce your risk of developing osteoporosis. Additionally, making smart choices about nutrition and lifestyle will allow for living a full, productive, and healthy life while you face the challenges of CRPS.

ooooo

Frozen Shoulder (Adhesive Capsulitis)

Frozen shoulder is a condition where a shoulder becomes very painful and stiff. Movements of the shoulder become reduced, sometimes completely 'frozen'. It is thought to be due to scar-like tissue forming in the shoulder capsule. Without treatment, symptoms usually go, but this may take up to 2–3 years. Various treatments are used to ease pain and improve the movement of the shoulder.

What are the symptoms of frozen shoulder?
The typical symptoms are pain, stiffness, and limitation in the range of movement of a shoulder. The symptoms typically have three phases.
- **Phase one – the 'freezing', painful phase.** This typically lasts 2–9 months. The first symptom is usually pain. Stiffness and limitation in movement then also gradually build up. The pain is typically worse at night and when lying on the affected side.
- **Phase two – the 'frozen', stiff phase.** This typically lasts 4–12 months. Pain gradually eases but stiffness and limitation in movement can get worse. All movements of the shoulder are affected but the movement most severely affected is usually rotation of the arm outwards. The muscles around the shoulder may waste a bit as they are not used.
- **Phase three – the 'thawing', recovery phase.** This typically lasts 5–24 months. The stiffness gradually goes and movement gradually returns to normal or near normal.

Symptoms often interfere with everyday tasks, such as driving, dressing or sleeping. Even scratching your back or putting your hand in a rear pocket may become impossible. Work may be affected in some cases.

There is a great variation in the severity and length of symptoms. Untreated, on average the symptoms last 2–3 years in total before going. In some cases it is much less than this. In a minority of cases symptoms can last for several years.

Who gets frozen shoulder?
The cause is not clear. It is thought that some scar tissue forms in the shoulder capsule. The capsule is a thin tissue that covers and protects the shoulder joint. The scar tissue may cause the capsule to thicken, contract and limit the movement of the shoulder. The reason why the scar tissue forms is not known.

A frozen shoulder occasionally follows a shoulder injury, but this is not usual and most cases occur for no apparent reason.

Anti-inflammatory painkillers – For example, ibuprofen, diclofenac, naproxen, etc. One of these drugs is commonly prescribed to ease pain. There are many different brands. Therefore, if one does not suit another may be fine. Side effects sometimes occur with anti-inflammatory painkillers. Always read the leaflet that comes with the drug packet for a full list of cautions and possible side effects.

Ordinary Painkillers – Paracetamol or codeine may be an option if anti-inflammatory painkillers do not suit. These do not have any anti-inflammatory action but are good painkillers. Constipation is a common side-effect from codeine. You can take painkillers in addition to other treatments.

Shoulder exercises – These are commonly advised. The aim is to keep the shoulder from 'stiffening up', and to keep movement as full as possible. For most benefit, it is important to do the exercises regularly, as instructed by a doctor or physiotherapist.

Physiotherapy – Many people are referred to a physiotherapist who can give expert advice on the best exercises to use. Also, they may try other pain relieving techniques such as heat, cold, Transcutaneous Electrical Nerve Stimulator (TENS) machines, etc.

A steroid injection – An injection into, or near to, the shoulder joint brings good relief of symptoms for several weeks in some cases. Steroids reduce inflammation. It is not a 'cure' as symptoms tend to gradually return, but many people welcome the relief that a steroid injection can bring.

Nerve block – This is a technique that a specialist may try. This is an injection to block the nerves that send pain messages from the shoulder. Like a steroid injection, it often eases symptoms for a while, but is not usually a cure.

Hydrodistension – Again this is a technique that a specialist may try. This is a procedure where the joint space is expanded (distended) by injecting a liquid. In one study, saline (salt water) mixed with a steroid injected into the painful shoulder improved symptoms in a number of cases.

Surgery – An operation is sometimes considered if other treatments do not help. Techniques that are used include:
- Manipulation. This is a procedure where the shoulder is moved around by the surgeon while you are under anaesthetic.
- Arthroscopic capsular release. This is a relatively small operation done as 'keyhole' surgery. It is often done as a day-case procedure. In this procedure the tight capsule of the joint is released with a special probe. One recent research study showed that this procedure gave about an 8 in 10 chance of greatly improving symptoms. Because of the encouraging results of this research study, it may become a more popular treatment.

ooooo

Historical References

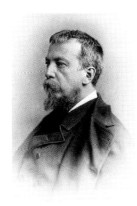

Weir Mitchell of Philadelphia
1829–1914

American neurology really began during the Civil War, chiefly through the work of S. Weir Mitchell and William A. Hammond. Appointed as surgeon-general of the U.S. Army Medical Department in 1862, Hammond undertook many projects and reforms, including the establishment of Turner's Lane Hospital outside of Philadelphia. In that 400-bed hospital devoted exclusively to the care of soldiers with neurologic disorders, Mitchell distinguished himself as a clinician with powers of meticulous observation.

Born in Philadelphia in 1821, Mitchell attended the University of Pennsylvania and graduated from Jefferson Medical College in 1850 at age 21. He recalled later, "I made up my mind that by thirty-five I should have a chair in one or the other of the two great schools", a wish that was frustrated all his life. Mitchell was a general practitioner, conducting some research in toxicology, when the Civil War began. His interest in neurologic disorders became evident to his friend Hammond, who appointed him to a small army hospital in Philadelphia devoted to neurologic patients. After the battle of Gettysburg, the hospital was moved to a larger building on Turner's Lane to accommodate the wounded.

With the collaboration of George R. Morehouse and William W. Keen, Mitchell published in 1864 the classic book **Gunshot Wounds and Other Injuries of the Nerves**. They reported their first 18 months experience, including a description of the clinical syndrome Mitchell later termed 'causalgia', a painful condition following injury to a large peripheral nerve. An expanded book written solely by Mitchell, **Injuries of the Nerves and**

Their Consequences, was published in 1872. His son, John Kearsley Mitchell, described **Remote Consequences of Injuries to Nerves** in 1895, reporting a follow-up of 20 of the original patients. Mitchell and his colleagues recognized the opportunity afforded by Turner's Lane Hospital, writing, "Never before in medical history has there been collected for study and treatment so remarkable a series of nerve injuries" (Mitchell, 1905). Their method of study began with an accurate account of each patient's symptoms and signs:

Keen, Morehouse, and I worked on at notetaking often as late as 12 or 1 at night, and when we got through walked home, talking over our cases. … The cases were of amazing interest. Here at one time were eighty epileptics, and every kind of nerve wound, palsies, choreas, stump disorders. (Mitchell, 1905)

Causalgia was observed in numerous soldiers at Turner's Lane Hospital. The pain was described as an intense, diffuse, burning sensation, subject to exacerbation by stimuli, mental as well as physical. Treatment at the time included water dressings and morphine injections. Mitchell (1872) described causalgia as "the most terrible of all the tortures which a nerve wound may inflict". He was a master of clinical case descriptions, and the following is an account of a case of causalgia in a Union soldier wounded in battle:

H., aged thirty-nine, New York, was shot July 2, 1863, through the inner edge of the right biceps, half an inch above the internal condyle of the humerus; the ball passed backward and downward. The musket fell from his left hand, and the right, grasping the rod, was twisted towards the chest and bent at the elbow. He walked to the rear. He cannot tell how much motion was lost, but he knows that he had instant pain in the median distribution, with tenderness of the palm, even on the first day, and a sense of numbness. My notes described him on entering our wards as presenting the following symptoms: the temperature of the two palms is alike. The back of the hand looks as usual, but the skin of the palm is delicate and thin, and without eruption. The joints of the fingers are swollen, and the hand secretes freely a sour, ill-smelling sweat. The pain is, in the first place, neuralgic, and darting down the median nerve track into the fingers; while in the second place, there is burning in the palm and up the anterior face of the fingers.
Pressure on the cicatrix gave no pain, but the median nerve below that point was tender, and pressure upon it caused pain in the hand. There was slight want of tactile sensibility in the median distribution in the hand, but the parts receiving the ulnar

nerve presented no sign of injury. The hyperesthesia of the palm was excessive, so that even to blow on it seemed to give pain. He kept it wrapped up and wet, but could not endure to pour water on to the palm, preferring to wet the dorsum of the hand and allow the fluid to run around, so as by degrees to soak the palm. After a few weeks of this torment he became so sensitive that the rustle of a paper or of a woman's dress, the sound of feet, the noise of a band, all appeared to increase his pain. His countenance at this time was worn, pinched, anaemic, his temper irritable, and his manner so odd that some of the attendants believed him insane. When questioned as to his condition he assured me that every strong moral emotion made him worse,–anger or disappointment expressing themselves cruelly in the aching limb. (Mitchell, 1872)

After the Civil War, Mitchell limited his practice to consultations in neurologic disease, for his reputation was wide and his service in demand. He made much of his living in psychiatry, however, with a particular interest in the treatment of hysteria in women. Friend of Oliver Wendell Holmes, William Osler, William James, and Walt Whitman, Mitchell made his mark in literature as well as medicine, as author of novels, short stories, and poems. In urging him to visit Boston, Holmes wrote to Mitchell, "I am lonely. You are the only friend of distinction left to me."

Charles Stewart Roberts
Copyright © 1990 Butterworth Publishers
From Clinical Methods. The History, Physical and Laboratory Examinations. Third Edition H. Kenneth Walker, W. Dallas Hall. J. Willis Hurst. Butterworths.

References:
- Burr AR. Weir Mitchell, his life and letters. New York: Duffield, 1929.
- Mitchell SW. Injuries of nerves and their consequences. Philadelphia: J. B. Lippincott, 1872.
- Mitchell SW. Some personal recollections of the Civil War. Trans Coll Phys Phila. 1905; 27: 87–94.

ooooo

Occupational Therapy

Some of the women who played a significant role in its creation and development in the United Kingdom.

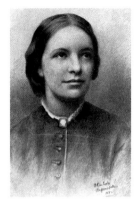

Octavia Hill
1838–1912

This remarkable woman can lay claim to having founded amongst others, the National Trust, the modern concepts of social work and housing associations, the Green Belt around London and the Army Cadet movement. Octavia believed passionately that 'the poor should never be denied beauty, simply through accident of birth'; and she therefore encouraged music, art and drama in all her projects. Perhaps above all she believed in the life-enhancing virtues of 'pure earth, clean air and blue sky'.

Her strong connection with occupational therapy comes through her influence on the young Elizabeth Casson who she employed to manage Red Cross Community Hall where the 'tired inhabitants of Southwark' enjoyed theatrical performances, concerts and poetry readings and the haven of Red Cross Garden, one of Octavia's 'open air sitting rooms', with pond, fountain, meandering paths, benches and flowers. Recently restored to its Victorian glory.

Picture Credit – Portrait Octavia Hill
Wellcome Library London

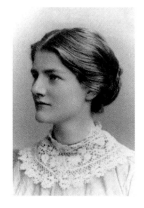

DR. ELIZABETH CASSON OBE MD DPM
1881–1954

Born in Denbigh, North Wales, she later moved to London with her musical and artistic family. From 1908 to 1913, she worked under Octavia Hill at Red Cross Hall, Southwark before deciding to train as a doctor and ultimately becoming an eminent psychiatrist and winner of the Gaskell Prize in 1927.

In 1929 she established her own residential clinic in Bristol, Dorset House, for 'women with mental disorders', and worked as its medical director. It was here in 1930 that she founded the first school of Occupational Therapy in the UK, Dorset House, The Promenade, Clifton.

Dr. Casson's plan for Dorset House was in her words:
"… to form a community where every individual was encouraged to feel that she had a real object; for a patient the object was to get well and go out to a worth-while life; for a member of the staff it was to serve others with all the talents she possessed; for a student, to develop all her capacities for her life as an Occupational Therapist and to find the individual job that only she could do."

She described a motivating incident:
"When I first qualified as a doctor … I found it very difficult to get used to the atmosphere of bored idleness in the day rooms of the hospital. Then, one Monday morning, when I arrived at the women's wards, I found the atmosphere had completely changed and realised that preparations for Christmas decorations had begun. The ward sisters had produced coloured tissue paper and bare branches, and all the patients were working happily in groups making flowers and leaves and using all their artistic talents with real interest and pleasure. I knew from that moment that such occupation was an integral part of treatment and must be provided."

She later (circa 1929) wrote:

"Occupational Therapy is a new healing method which is working such miracles with the mentally disordered and the victims of long and tedious convalescence."

The first Principal at Dorset House School of Occupational Therapy was Constance Tebbit (later Owens) who returned from training as an occupational therapist in Philadelphia to take up her post. She later went on to set up the Liverpool School of Occupational Therapy.

In 1951 Dr. Casson was awarded the OBE for her work and was elected an Honorary Fellow of the World Federation of Occupational Therapists. In 1973 the Dr. Elizabeth Casson annual memorial lecture was established and the Elizabeth Casson rose was created to mark the 50th anniversary of her death and launched at Chelsea Flower Show in 2005.

Margaret Barr Fulton MBE 1900–1989

In 1925 Peg Fulton, as she was known, became the first occupational therapist to work in the United Kingdom. She qualified at the Philadelphia School in the United States and was appointed to the Aberdeen Royal Hospital for mental patients where she worked until her retirement in 1963. During that time, she gained an international reputation for her department and for her part in the development of both the Scottish Association (SAOT) and the World Federation of Occupational Therapists (WFOT).

Picture Credit – Portrait Elizabeth Casson aged 21:
Image from the Dorset House Archive, Oxford Brookes University Library. Reproduced by permission of the Elizabeth Casson Trust.

Elizabeth Casson Quotes: The College of Occupational Therapists 2004, Elizabeth Casson OBE MD DPM 1881–1954. London, The College of Occupational Therapists

ooooo

The origins and history of the Alexander Technique

"You translate everything, whether physical or mental or spiritual, into muscular tension."

F.M. Alexander

"Mr. Alexander has done a service to the subject [of the study of reflex and voluntary movement] by insistently treating each act as involving the whole integrated individual, the whole psychophysical man. To take a step is an affair, not of this or that limb solely, but of the total neuromuscular activity of the moment, not least of the head and neck."

Sir Charles Sherrington 1857–1952
Neurophysiologist, Nobel Prize for Medicine 1932

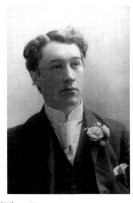

Frederick Matthias Alexander
1869–1955

The Beginning

The Alexander Technique was first developed in the 1890s by an Australian named Frederick Matthias Alexander. As a young and promising actor, Alexander faced a problem which risked ending his career – his voice would become increasingly hoarse during performances, until he could barely produce any sound at all. He consulted doctors, but they could not diagnose any specific disease or cause of the hoarseness. If there were no clear medical cause for his problem, Alexander reasoned that he might be doing something wrong when reciting, leading him to strain or 'misuse' his own vocal organs. As his only resort was self-help, he decided to observe his way of speaking and reciting to see whether he could spot anything unusual and find a solution.

Health and Performance

What emerged from this experiment of several years was more than just a vocal technique. Alexander gradually realised that the functioning of the voice depended on the correct balance of tension in his entire neuromuscular system, from head to toe. Alexander developed his technique to encourage and maintain this balance through conscious attention and control: a technique which has become applicable to a wide range of problems and aims. In short, this balance was extremely important for overall coordination and many other functions, such as breathing, posture, freedom of the joints in moving the whole body, using the arms and hands for skilled activities, staying calm under pressure, and maintaining good overall health.

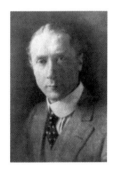

F.M. Alexander
in 1910

Gradually, as others noticed improved health and performance, he began to show his technique to those who came to him for help. From about 1894 onward, he had flourishing practices in Melbourne, and later in Sydney, until this teaching became his main occupation. A number of doctors referred patients to him, including Charles Bage, the Melbourne doctor he had once consulted for his voice trouble; actors also flocked to him for help. In 1904, in order to gain more recognition for his Technique, and prompted by his friend JW Steward MacKay, an eminent Sidney surgeon, he moved to London, where he worked until his death in 1955.

Recognition

In London, Alexander's reputation grew rapidly. One of his earliest acquaintances and pupils was Sir Henry Irving, considered the greatest Shakespearean actor of his time. Many doctors, including Peter MacDonald, later to become chairman of the BMA, endorsed his work and sent patients to him. In 1939, a group of physicians wrote to the **British Medical Journal** urging that Alexander's principles be included in medical training. Eminent thinkers who went to Alexander included George Bernard Shaw and Aldous Huxley. A number of scientists also endorsed his method, recognising that Alexander's practical observations were consistent with scientific discoveries in neurology and physiology. The most eminent of these was Sir Charles Sherrington, today considered the father of modern neurology. With its wide application,

Alexander's technique drew people from all walks of life, including politics (Sir Stafford Cripps and Lord Lytton), religion (William Temple, Archbishop of Canterbury), education (Esther Lawrence, principal of the Froebel Institute) and business (Joseph Rowntree).

Education

Alexander also spent a good deal of time during and between the two world wars in the USA, where he met and gave lessons to the philosopher John Dewey, an eminent innovator in theories about education. Dewey asserted that effective learning must be based on first-hand experience; he demonstrated his support and enthusiasm for Alexander's work by writing the prefaces to three of Alexander's books. Alexander believed it was important to incorporate his technique into the field of education to prevent problems and to improve learning at an early stage. In 1924, after Alexander worked successfully

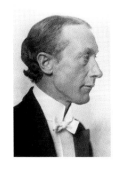

F.M. Alexander
in 1920

with a child with educational learning problems, some of his pupils asked to send their children to him for lessons. He then founded the 'Little School' in London, helped by two of his assistants, Ethel Webb and Irene Tasker, who had been trained as school teachers by Maria Montessori in Italy. In the school, children were encouraged to maintain optimal coordination in all their activities, while following their academic lessons. The children were evacuated to the USA during the Second World War but, sadly, it proved too difficult to re-establish the school in London in the immediate aftermath of the war.

Passing on the Technique

Up to the 1930s, Alexander taught his technique to pupils solely as a means of their helping themselves. A few of his keenest pupils gradually became assistants and teachers in their own right by apprenticeship. Then, in 1931, Alexander opened a formal teacher training course, so that an entire group of students could learn the skills needed to teach the Technique to others. He kept his three-year training courses running until his death at the age of 86. In 1958, three years after his death, his graduates founded the Society of Teachers of the Alexander Technique (STAT), to preserve and continue the work according to the standards Alexander had created and training methods have continued to evolve.

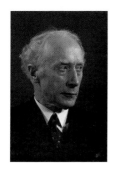

F.M. Alexander
in 1941

That the Alexander Technique has endured, and that there are now over 2500 teachers throughout the world, is indicative of its scope beyond the problems or talent of one charismatic person; the Technique is founded on principles and skills which can apply to anyone. People have come to the United Kingdom from around the world to study the Technique, while professional societies and teacher training courses affiliated to STAT have been established in 14 other countries. The Technique is taught in all the major performing arts colleges in the United Kingdom, and has also been introduced in a number of elementary and secondary schools.

A number of small research studies have been undertaken to study the Alexander Technique as applied to various medical problems, and the first large scale study on the Alexander Technique and back pain, at the University of Southampton, began its trial phase in 2002.

"Instead of feeling one's body to be an aggregation of ill-fitting parts full of friction and dead weights pulling this way and that, so as to render mere existence in itself exhausting, the body becomes a coordinated and living whole, composed of well-fitting and truly articulated parts."

Sir Stafford Cripps
Former Chancellor of the Exchequeur

"When an investigation comes to be made, it will be found that every single thing we are doing in this work is exactly what happens in Nature where the conditions are right, the difference being that we are learning to do it consciously."

F.M. Alexander

ooooo

The Origins of Osteopathy

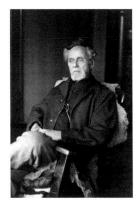

Andrew Taylor Still
1828–1917

Andrew Taylor Still, founder of Osteopathy, was a medical doctor in America's Midwest. He had been in practice ten years when, in a devastating two-week period, he lost three of his own children and an adopted girl during an outbreak of meningitis. Heartbroken and utterly disillusioned at the inefficacy of the drugs of the day, he embarked on a quest to find a better way of practising medicine.

Going back to first principles – anatomy and physiology – he founded Osteopathy in 1874 on the premise that every cell of the body is constantly striving to express perfect health. Dr. Still determined that instead of trying to control the physiological changes called disease, with drugs, the role of the doctor should be to create the right conditions for the body to heal itself. He built Osteopathy on the principle that, for their normal function, cells require an uninterrupted supply of oxygen and nutrients, removal of the waste products of cellular metabolism, and regulation of the circulation by the nervous system. This will only occur efficiently, he discovered through long experience in practice, when the structure of the body is free from mechanical derangement.

Through cultivating his sense of touch and developing methods of correcting joint and soft tissue strains, he discovered that he had found a system of treatment that was both curative and preventative, and applicable to virtually every condition. He rapidly gained a reputation for tackling every disease he was presented with. Treat the cause, he would say, and the effect will disappear.

Still founded the first Osteopathic school in the small town of Kirksville, Missouri in 1892. Known affectionately as the 'old doctor', within five years he had trained 500 Osteopaths (including several of his own children), and at any one time there were 500 patients lodged in the town, receiving treatment at the infirmary. This enormous success was built on his reputation alone, without any advertising. By the year of his death, Still had trained over 6,000 Osteopaths. In that same year, one of his students, a Scot named J Martin Littlejohn, opened the UK's first Osteopathic school, the British School of Osteopathy, in London.

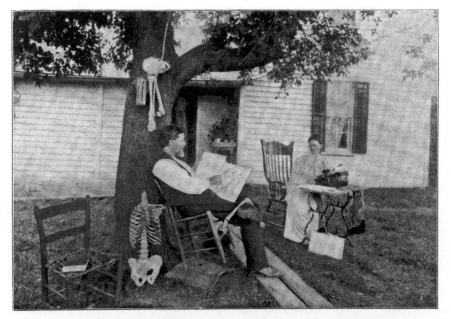

DR. A. T. STILL AND MRS. ANNIE MORRIS, HIS AMANUENSIS.

Mrs. Morris's residence in the background, where Dr. Still studied many of the problems of Osteopathy,

Wellcome Library London

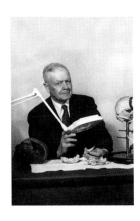

WILLIAM GARNER SUTHERLAND
1873–1954

William Garner Sutherland DO had the opportunity to study with Dr. Andrew Taylor Still, the founder of the science of Osteopathy. In his teaching, Dr. Still always emphasised the design for motion in the articulations of the bones.

One day in 1899, during Sutherland's senior year at the American School of Osteopathy, he viewed a specially prepared and mounted skull. At that moment, Sutherland experienced a flash of insight which saw the articulation of the spheno-squamous suture as a design for motion that implied a respiratory mechanism, 'like the gills of a fish'. Given the statements in anatomical texts that the sutures of the cranium ossify in the adult, he had much scepticism and reservation about his own insight for years. During his in-depth studies in the following years, Dr. Sutherland had to confront the fact of a mobility that has no muscular agencies to account for the motion.

This kind of study of the mechanics of articular mechanisms of the living human body led him to recognise powers within his patients which could resolve problems and heal strains. Based on what he learned from his patients, Dr. Sutherland developed many ways of practising Osteopathy. He considered that he was utilising a profound science which just kept unfolding its truths. Dr. Sutherland often said in his lectures that if you understand the mechanism, the treatment is simple.

From Teachings in the Science of Osteopathy, edited by Anne L Wales DO, Sutherland Cranial Teaching Foundation, ISBN 0-915801-26-4.

235

"The goal of an Osteopathic treatment is to affect a more efficient interchange between all the fluids of the body and across all their tissue interfaces."

William G. Sutherland, D.O.

"Osteopathy is a science with possibilities as great as the magnitude of the heavens. It is a science dealing with the natural forces of the body. We work as Osteopaths with the traditional principle in mind that the tendency in the patient's body is always toward the normal. There is much to discover in the science of Osteopathy by working with the forces within that manifest the healing processes. These forces within the patient are greater than any blind force that can safely be brought to bear from without."

William Garner Sutherland, D.O., D.Sc. (hon.)

Reprinted By kind permission of Sutherland Cranial Teaching Foundation. Photograph of William Garner Sutherland Reprinted By Kind Permission of Sutherland Cranial Teaching Foundation.

ooooo

Dr. Shan-Chi Ko – Collateral Meridian Therapy

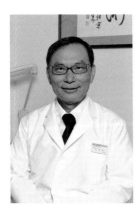

Dr. Shan-Chi Ko

Dr. Shan-Chi Ko was born in Taiwan. After graduating from the medical school at Japan's National Kagoshima University, Dr. Ko worked at the Department of Anesthesiology and ICU at Japan's Kyushu University Hospital and the Radiology Department at National Kyushu Cancer Center. From 1985 through 2001, he established two clinics in Fukuoka and Koga where he served as an internist.

Throughout his career as a physician, Dr. Ko searched for different ways to treat pain. Not content with the treatments available in today's conventional medicine, Dr. Ko studied Acupuncture at Shanghai University of Traditional Chinese Medicine and Pharmacology. After returning to Japan, he devoted himself to the pursuit of a more effective pain treatment. Over the next seven years, and with more than 7500 clinical case studies, he developed a new theory for treating pain: By stimulating two pressure points, most local pains can be noticeably reduced almost immediately. (This theory was later refined to treat CNS-related symptoms as well.) His theory was published in the Shanghai Journal of Acupuncture and Moxibustion (2001, 6th Issue). In February 2002, Dr. Ko publicly presented 'New Dimension in Pain Therapy: Distant Point Immediate-Effect Press Therapy', which he later named 'Collateral Meridian Therapy' (CMT). His presentation was well received by the 120 doctors in attendance.

History of CMT and Enrac

Since CMT was first presented in Tokyo in 2002, the active research and application of CMT in Japan and Taiwan have created a noticeable impact in the academic, medical, and clinical sectors of pain relief. CMT began gaining notice in the US medical community in 2006.

2002.02   Dr. Ko's theory of Collateral Meridian Therapy (CMT) was published for the first time in Tokyo.

2002.06   Painless Ginza Clinic, the first clinic in Japan specializing in treating intractable pain, was established in Tokyo.

2002.10   The Enrac® Ko Medicine Medical Team of Japan was established.

2003.08   The theory of CMT was presented in Taiwan for the first time a the Center of Medical Education, Taipei Veteran General Hospital.

2003.12   Enrac® Medical Society of Japan, Taiwan office, was established.

2006.05   The Enrac® Medical Society of Taiwan was established.

2006.06   The Medical School of Kitasato University, Japan, held a CMT workshop.

2006.09   Dr. Ko's book, **There Is No Pain that Cannot Be Cured**, was published in Taiwan.

2006.09   Enrac® Ko Medicine Medical Team of Taiwan was established.

2006.11   The first CMT seminar in the USA was held at Duke University Medical Center.

2007.01   Dr. Ko was invited by WFATT to speak at the World Congress on Sports Injury Prevention Conference. Tokyo, Japan

2007.04   Enrac USA was established.

2008.05   13th International Pain Clinic Congress The 46th Scientific Meeting of the Korean Pain Society Topic: New Five Dimensional Pain Treatment – Enrac CMT

ooooo

Contacts

For Anatomical Charts and Study Guides visit The Anatomical Chart Company Skokie, IL, USA at **www.anatomical.com**

For those not online the charts are available in larger academic bookshops.

ooooo

For the Orthopaedic V Shaped Support Pillow (page 37) contact your local Argos Store.

ooooo

Patterson Medical Ltd.

Tel: 08444 124 330
Fax: 08448 730 100
homecraft.sales@patterson-medical.com

www.homecraft-rolyan.com
www.mobilisrolyan.com

THANKS

To All my friends
Christian, Mimi, Elizabeth and Jeff, Rob and Shal, May and Mathew, Pam and Victor, Sharif, Bonita, Agnes, Ann W, Vanessa L, Barbara, Rex, Oisin, Kenny R and Elaine and David who supported me unconditionally, emotionally and financially through a traumatic year and then some.

To The doctors and health care professionals
Some names are changed for legal reasons
Dr. Morris, whose speedy referral was the first step in saving my hand. The Consultant Ms AS whose sure appraisal of the situation ensured I could begin positive work on recovery and who later installed plates in both wrists after my second accident. To Terry (Hand Therapist) who launched that recovery and whose excellent knowledge of her job informed Elizabeth and myself about what we could do at home to back up what happened in treatment. To Amy who introduced me to the fantastic mirror work. To Lizzy whose Alexander Technique reminded me to breathe and be conscious of my whole body posture and practise at home. To Dr. Zhu, who brought down the turgid swelling in my hand with his superb Acupuncture. Marilena who massaged and taught me pain meditation and whose herbs and tinctures soothed my frazzled nerves. Demian, who gave me a whole new view on what I was experiencing and introduced me to a number of ideas to calm my nerves. Joseph (Occupational Therapist) who restored my faith in the NHS and always made me feel as though he genuinely cared whether I recovered or not. To the extraordinary Dr. Ko and Dr. Wang who took away some of the overwhelming and constant crippling pain I had experienced for seven months. To all at Enrac who made my stay in Taiwan so good.

To Mr R who assessed my shoulder and assured me that the route I had chosen was effective and showed genuine interest in the alternative and complementary methods I had accessed. Finally to the extraordinary Mr Lakhani, whose excellent Osteopathy finally gave relief to my shoulder and facilitated the unlocking of my wrist and the shedding of my oedema glove and ridding me once and for all of the residual pain.

Thank you, thank you, thank you.